UNTIL THERE IS A CURE
The Latest and Greatest in Diabetes Self-Care

Gary Scheiner, MS, CDE

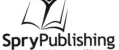

SpryPublishing
ideas to life

This edition is published by
Spry Publishing LLC
2500 South State Street
Ann Arbor, MI 48104 USA

Printed and bound in the United States of America.

10 9 8 7 6 5 4 3 2 1

Library of Congress Control Number: 2012955507

Paperback ISBN: 978-1-938170-10-2
E-book ISBN: 978-1-938170-13-3

Disclaimer: Spry Publishing LLC does not assume responsibility
for the contents or opinions expressed herein. Although every precaution
is taken to ensure that information is accurate as of the date of
publication, differences of opinion exist. The opinions expressed herein
are those of the author and do not necessarily reflect the views of
the publisher. The information contained in this book is not intended
to replace professional advisement of an individual's doctor
prior to beginning or changing an individual's course of treatment.

Contents

Until There Is a Cure ...

I never used to believe in that saying, "The more things change, the more they stay the same." Then I entered the diabetes field.

This book is all about keeping pace with the changes —changing technology, changing therapies, changing approaches to diabetes management. Basically the information provided here will help you take advantage of what's "new and improved," and ultimately make your diabetes control a little bit better and living with this chronic condition a little bit easier.

With changes taking place all around us, what exactly has stayed the same? For starters, the goal of diabetes management is roughly the same: to manage blood sugar as effectively as possible so that it does not keep us from enjoying life to the fullest. The emphasis on self-management hasn't really changed. Experts recognize that diabetes is the type of condition that involves countless choices and decisions on the part of the patient on a daily basis. To expect your doctor or nurse to be there all the time is a pipedream. We, as people with diabetes, must educate ourselves and obtain and use the necessary tools to manage effectively.

One other constant through the years is hope. We all hope that doing the right things will produce the desired results. We also hope for a cure. Back in 1985 when I was diagnosed with type 1 diabetes in a Texas town called Sugarland (God's honest truth!), my endocrinologist tried to convince me how lucky I was to be diagnosed when I was.

"We've come a long way in recent years," he said. "The way research is going, in 5 or 10 years, your diabetes will probably be cured."

That was more than 25 years ago. Still no cure, but people are still saying, "In 5 or 10 years ... we'll have a cure." Although there is some very promising research taking place, I'm not one to put my eggs in that basket. My personal goal, and what I emphasize to my patients, is to take the best possible care of their diabetes here and now. When a cure does finally come along—and it will—I want to be in the best of health and have no regrets about the effort I put in.

Today, I can look back at the way diabetes was treated when I was diagnosed and say, "Man, those were the Stone Ages!" But you know what? Five or ten years from now, I'll probably look back to today and think the very same thing. At least I hope so.

WHY MANAGE?

Whether you've had diabetes for a month or a millennium, you know that managing it takes work. There are sacrifices to be made, expenses involved, and mental and physical energy that you'd probably rather use on something a bit more fun. If you're going to put the work in, you deserve to get something for it. Here's a quick overview of what you stand to gain.

Immediate Benefits
- **Increased Energy** Elevated blood glucose reduces energy levels. Fuel that should be available to your muscles is floating around in the bloodstream instead. This tends to cause sleepiness and sluggishness. As soon as glucose levels return to normal, energy levels usually improve.
- **More Restful Sleep** The quality of sleep is affected by poor glucose control. If your glucose is high enough, you might wake up several times during the night to run to the bathroom. Low glucose will probably wake you as well. Most people with diabetes report feeling better rested when glucose levels are well controlled through the night.
- **Improved Physical Performance** Glucose control has an immediate effect on your physical abilities. Elevated glucose can reduce your strength, flexibility, speed, stamina, and endurance. Low sugar levels impair coordination and muscle function. When glucose levels are near normal, your energy and physical performance can be maximized.
- **Appetite Reduction** Ever feel like there is no end to your hunger? High glucose may be to blame. If not enough sugar is getting into your body's cells, hunger is going to increase. Controlling glucose levels is a good way to keep your appetite in check.

- **Brain Power** High and low glucose limits our ability to focus, remember, perform complex tasks, and be creative. Wide variations in blood sugar levels, such as "rises and falls" that occur after meals, have also been shown to hinder intellectual function. Improving your glucose control will make it easier for your brain to operate at its best. There is also evidence that people with uncontrolled diabetes have a higher incidence of Alzheimer's disease.

- **Stable Moods/Emotions** The brain is also responsible for maintaining our emotional balance. Moods often change along with our blood sugars. High glucose levels can make us impatient, irritable, and generally negative. Achieving near-normal blood sugars and keeping them there can go a long way toward improving your mood and emotional stability.

- **Fewer Sick Days** Infection-causing bacteria and viruses thrive on glucose. When sugar levels are up, we become virtual breeding grounds for infection. Everything from common colds and sinus infections to flu and vaginal yeast infections are less common when blood sugars are well controlled.

- **Healthier Skin and Gums** Both the skin and gums are affected quickly by elevated glucose levels. Since skin is influenced by our level of hydration, when blood sugars are high, skin tends to become dry and cracked. And bacteria that live below the gum line grow quickly when exposed to high sugar levels in our blood vessels. These bacteria then form plaque at an accelerated rate, contributing to bleeding gums and loose teeth.

Controlling your diabetes will help cut back on plaque buildup immediately.

- **Personal Safety** If you drive a car, operate power equipment, play a sport, or just walk across the street, uncontrolled blood sugar can put you at risk. High glucose can cause sleepiness and slow reaction times (a recipe for disaster when driving). And the opposite extreme, hypoglycemia (low blood sugar) will always cause some degree of mental impairment. Decision-making and judgment will be off. Coordination suffers and trembling can occur. To keep yourself and those around you safe, blood sugar must be managed properly.
- **Predictable Periods** Women with near-normal HbA1c levels (a measurement of average glucose levels over several months) tend to have more regular menstrual cycles than women with an elevated A1c. Blood glucose levels that are maintained at near-normal levels will minimize some of the negative symptoms associated with the menstrual cycle.

Long-Term Benefits

Glucose levels that are too high over a period of many years cause damage to virtually every important system of the body. Major long-term multi-center research projects have shown that tight glucose control reduces the risk of many long-term health problems. There are no guarantees, but odds are that if you manage your diabetes well, you can look forward to the following:

- **Healthy Eyes** Diabetic retinopathy is the leading cause of blindness among adults aged 20 to 74. Tight blood sugar control reduces the risk of retinopathy. Research has shown that every 1 percent reduction in HbA1c (30 mg/dl or 1.7 mmol/l reduction in average blood sugar) corresponds to a 30 percent reduction in the risk of developing retinopathy.

- **Healthy Kidneys** Uncontrolled diabetes is also the leading cause of kidney failure. Elevated blood sugar damages the tiny blood vessels (capillaries) that form and nourish the filters within the kidneys. As was the case with retinopathy, every 1 percent reduction in HbA1c produces a 30 percent reduction in the risk of kidney disease.

- **Ample Circulation** People with diabetes are two to four times more likely to develop heart disease and five times more likely to die from heart disease compared to people without diabetes. Besides the heart, a number of other body parts, such as the brain and leg muscles, require large amounts of oxygen and nutrients. Excessive amounts of sugar in the bloodstream contribute to atherosclerosis or thickening of the arteries. When blood vessels become clogged, bad things happen: heart attacks, strokes, and pain or cramping in the legs. Improving glucose control reduces the risk of blood vessel disease and facilitates adequate circulation to all parts of the body.

- **Proper Nerve Function** Our nervous system serves as the "wiring" for our bodies. The "autonomic" portion of our nervous system allows the brain to control behind-the-scenes functions such as heart rate, digestion, and sexual function. The "peripheral" portion controls movements and provides sensation from the extremities.

Elevated blood sugar causes two problems for nerves: it interferes with their blood supply and energy metabolism is altered causing the nerves to swell and lose their protective coating.

Sixty to seventy percent of people with diabetes will develop some form of nerve damage in their lifetime. Nearly 50 percent of all men with diabetes develop erectile dysfunction (impotency), and 30 percent of people with diabetes suffer from delayed digestion (gastroparesis). Postural hypotension (low blood pressure upon sitting or standing) is twice as common in people with diabetes. Damage to peripheral nerves can produce tingling or numbness. As it progresses, constant and sometimes severe pain can develop. Tight blood sugar control is an effective means for preventing all forms of neuropathy. And for those with existing neuropathy, the symptoms may improve as blood sugar levels improve.

- **Fit Feet** Loss of protective nerve sensation, combined with poor circulation, can lead to serious foot infections and deformities. Each year, more than 70,000 people with diabetes require lower-limb amputations—that's more than all other causes combined. Tight blood sugar control helps to preserve healthy nerve function and blood flow to the feet. Lowering blood sugar levels also reduces the risk for infection.
- **A Sound Mind** Alzheimer's disease is a progressive and fatal illness that destroys brain cells, causing problems with memory, thinking, and behavior. Today, it is the sixth-leading cause of death in the United States, affecting

more than 5 million Americans. Damaged blood vessels in the brain are believed to play a role in the development of Alzheimer's. Uncontrolled diabetes, which contributes to blood vessel damage, greatly increases the risk of Alzheimer's disease. Tight blood sugar control can reduce the risk of Alzheimer's to that of the non-diabetic population.

- **Flexible Joints** Joint mobility problems, including frozen shoulder, trigger fingers, and clawed hands, affect approximately 20 percent of people with diabetes. Excess sugar sticks to collagen, a protein found in bones, cartilage, and connective tissue throughout the body. This keeps joints from moving smoothly through the full range of motion and can also cause pain in the joints. Keeping blood sugar levels near normal reduces the risk of joint mobility problems. If you already have limited range of motion, lowering your blood sugar may help to improve your range of motion and limit the pain associated with stiff joints.

- **Good Mental Health** Blood sugar levels have a direct effect on mental well-being. Depression is three times more common in adults with diabetes than in the general population. Since depression is often biochemical in nature, elevated sugar levels in the fluid surrounding the brain may play a role. In addition, developing complications from diabetes can instill a feeling of helplessness, which is known to contribute to depression. Research has shown that when people with diabetes lower their blood ugar levels, they report a higher overall quality of life.

- **Successful Pregnancy** Women with diabetes face a number of potential risks involving childbirth, including fetal abnormalities and deliveries complicated by having a large baby. But don't despair. Women who manage their diabetes tightly during pregnancy can have healthy babies with success equal to women without diabetes.

MANAGEMENT OBJECTIVES

If our ultimate goal in managing diabetes is to live a long, healthy, high-quality life, we really should discuss what is meant by "management."

I define quality diabetes management as achieving the lowest possible HbA1c (defined below) without frequent or severe episodes of hypoglycemia. In other words, a decent average blood sugar and not too much bouncing around. Occasional, mild episodes of hypoglycemia are acceptable and not all that dangerous for most people. Once low blood sugars become too frequent (more than two or three a week) or severe (causing accidents, seizures, or loss of consciousness), it will be necessary to ease up or look for better ways to manage on a daily basis. Likewise, a mild rise in blood sugar after eating is acceptable, but huge spikes are not. Also, diabetes should not dominate your life. If you put more time and energy into taking care of your diabetes than you put into your family, work, or social life, something needs to change.

We also need to establish measurable objectives for assessing blood sugar control. In other words, what are some of our numeric targets?

As we've mentioned briefly, one of the numbers to consider is the hemoglobin A1c (also called a "glycosylated hemoglobin" or simply "A1c"). The A1c reflects the average glucose level for the past 2 to 3 months. The A1c is important because it correlates with the risk of long-term complications, such as eye, kidney, nerve, and blood vessel diseases. To convert your A1c into an average glucose (and vice versa), use the formulas below:

Avg Blood Glucose (in mg/dl) = (A1c x 28.7) - 46.7
Avg Blood Glucose (in mmol/l) = (A1c x 1.59) - 2.59
and in reverse:
A1c = (Avg BG (in mg/dl) + 46.7) / 28.7
A1c = (Avg BG (in mmol/l) + 2.59) / 1.59

Target ranges should be individualized based on your needs and capabilities. A "normal" or "nondiabetic" A1c is in the range of 4 to 6 percent, representing an average glucose of approximately 70 to 125 mg/dl (3.9–7.0 mmol/l). For most people with diabetes, particularly those who utilize an intensive insulin program, it is not possible to maintain an A1c in the "normal" range without experiencing excessive hypoglycemia or having to put far too much work into diabetes self-care. In most cases, efforts should be made to keep the A1c in the 6 to 7 percent range. Slightly higher targets may be sought by those who have hypoglycemia unawareness (those who don't receive low blood sugar warning symptoms) or those who have unstable heart disease, as well as those who work in high-risk professions. Slightly higher targets are also reasonable for young children who cannot detect or treat hypoglycemia independently. Lower targets may be sought by women during pregnancy, individuals planning for surgery, and those looking to slow or reverse existing complications.

Keep in mind that the A1c merely reflects an average. Our goal is to achieve stability as well. That means staying within your target glucose range as often as possible on a day-to-day basis.

Separate targets should be set for pre-meal glucose values versus the post-meal peak (1 to 1½ hours after finishing eating). In most cases, an A1c in the 6 to 7 percent range can be achieved by having the majority of pre-meal readings in the 70 to 160 mg/dl (4–9 mmol/l) range, and post-meal peaks below 180 mg/dl (10 mmol/l). See the table below for details:

Level of Control	A1c	Fasting and Pre-meal Acceptable Range mg/dl (mmol/l)	Post-Meal Acceptable Peak mg/dl (mmol/l)
Very tight	5–6 percent	60–140 (3.5–8)	<160 (<9)
Tight	6–7 percent	70–160 (4–9)	<180 (<10)
Average	7–8 percent	70–180 (4–10)	<200 (<11)
Loose	8–9 percent	80–200 (4.5–11)	<220 (<12)

The inclusion of post-meal targets is relatively new in the field of diabetes care. As research continues to point out the link between post-meal glucose "spikes" and the development of long-term and short-term complications, stronger emphasis is being placed on glucose stability. As you will see later in this book, new and innovative techniques have been developed to assess, measure, and ultimately manage post-meal glucose levels.

Don't expect to hit your pre-meal and post-meal targets every time you check your blood sugar! That would be like a basketball player never missing a shot or a baseball player never making an out. In general, it is desirable to "hit" your target at least 70 percent of the time, with fewer than 10 percent of your readings below the low end of your target range. But that's a long-term goal. Consider how often you're in the target range currently and work to improve on it. Every time you make a sensible program change or apply a new technique or technology, you should expect to see some improvement.

Another number to keep an eye on is called "standard deviation (SD)." This is a statistic generated by the glucose meter and continuous glucose monitoring via downloaded software. The standard deviation represents the amount of variability in your glucose values. A high SD means that you are having frequent and extreme high and low readings. A low SD indicates that your glucose values don't wander too far from your overall average. The lower your standard deviation, the better. Less glucose variability equates with a lower risk of long-term complications and better daily quality of life. An SD that is less than one-third of your average blood glucose is desirable. An SD that is more than half of your average indicates excessive variability in your control.

CHALLENGES TO INTENSIVE CONTROL

If only it was easy to hit those targets! Just consider what we're up against.

At any given time, there are approximately 5 grams of glucose in the bloodstream. That's it. Just a teaspoon's worth. That's what we're trying to maintain. Now consider these little tidbits:

- Our body can burn up glucose at a rapid rate (up to 2 grams per minute) during exercise.

- When we eat, dozens of grams of glucose can enter the bloodstream within an hour.
- We have a multitude of hormones, some produced on a daily or monthly cycle and some produced in response to environmental triggers, affecting our sensitivity to insulin as well as the liver's secretion of glucose into the bloodstream.
- Having diabetes means that we lack both insulin and amylin, a hormone that regulates the appearance of glucose in the bloodstream after meals. We also produce a glucose-raising hormone, glucagon, at inappropriate times.
- Whereas insulin secreted by the pancreas works very quickly (starts in seconds, peaks and finishes working in a few minutes), the fastest working, most rapid insulin we can take by injection starts working in 10 to 20 minutes and takes hours to peak and finish working. The majority of foods we eat raise the blood sugar significantly in less than an hour.

Now, think again about that teaspoon of glucose. Imagine yourself walking on a tightrope with that teaspoon balanced on the tip of your nose. Sugar is falling from the sky like rain. One of your arms is exercising feverishly, the other is feeding you carbohydrates. And all the while the audience is testing your balancing skills by throwing stress balls at your head. And all you have to do is keep that teaspoon of sugar from overflowing or spilling out. Every minute. Of every day.

That's why we can't be overly perfectionistic when it comes to blood sugar control. Set short-term, measurable, realistic goals, and don't lose sight of the big picture.

WHAT IT TAKES

Improving your diabetes management is just that ... doing better. Not perfect. Improvement requires the right attitude, education, and the ability to utilize the best tools and technologies the diabetes industry has to offer.

The Right Attitude

Nothing, and I mean nothing, takes place without proper motivation. You could have the top doctor in the country and the best tools and training the world has to offer. Without the right mental approach, it's all for naught.

Exactly where does managing diabetes rank in your set of personal priorities? If your diabetes is not well controlled, how will it affect you at work? At school? At home? At the gym? In bed? Although nobody would expect you to place your diabetes self-care above the immediate well-being of your family, it should hold a prominent place in your life. So be prepared to invest some time, energy, and funds into your diabetes management.

Persistence is another valuable trait. Over the course of your life with diabetes, there are sure to be many setbacks. Out-of-range readings. Undesired lab results. Lows at inappropriate times. And possibly the development of complications. When these things happen, it helps to live your diabetes life one day at a time. You can't change the past, so don't worry about what you did (or didn't do) yesterday. And you certainly can't live tomorrow until tomorrow. Every day represents an opportunity for a fresh start.

The right mental approach also includes a degree of

discipline, sticking to a plan even in the face of distraction and adversity. Maybe not all the time, but certainly most of the time. From my experience, people who are disciplined about things like keeping records, checking blood sugars, counting carbs, taking insulin before eating, and putting appropriate time frames between their meals and snacks (to avoid "grazing") tend to have better blood sugar control over the long term.

In terms of motivation, fear (of complications, for example) can be powerful, but it tends to be temporary. Long-term motivation stems from something personal that comes from within. Are you the type who is motivated by short-term challenges? Then play the numbers game and work on improving your control. Are you the type who will do things for others before you'll do them for yourself? If that's the case, serve as a role model for someone else or dedicate your diabetes self-care to someone special to you. Sometimes, motivation can come from a tangential goal, such as participating in an athletic event, having a baby, or simply being around long enough and healthy enough to dance at your grandkids' weddings. Whatever your motivation, latch onto it and use it to fuel your daily choices and activities.

Education

We've already established that self-management is a cornerstone of diabetes care. Not that we don't need ongoing medical guidance, but the "SELF" part means that each of us must have the know-how to take care of ourselves on a daily basis. If you've had diabetes for many years and think you learned all you need to know years ago, think again. The diabetes landscape is constantly changing. Ongoing education is essential if you're going to do the best job possible.

Sources of diabetes education include:
- Classes at local hospitals or clinics
- One-on-one sessions with Certified Diabetes Educators
- Conferences held by diabetes organizations
- Books on diabetes or related health topics
- Diabetes magazines, radio shows, and TV shows
- Newsletters from companies specializing in diabetes products or services
- Web sites sponsored by health-care organizations
- Web-based diabetes webinars
- Mobile device applications
- Online and face-to-face support groups

Some are free, some cost a little bit. Some you can access from home, some require a bit of travel. Regardless, the more you educate yourself, the better prepared you'll be to handle the challenges diabetes throws your way.

Tools and Technologies

Imagine trying to surf the Internet and watch streaming video on a computer that still uses a dial-up modem (can't you just hear those "Eeeeeyyoooo" sounds?). Or applying leeches to your body at the first signs of an infection? Trying to manage your diabetes using age-old equipment and methodology can be equally ineffective and frustrating.

The state of care in diabetes is changing rapidly. New medications and gadgets are being introduced all the time.

Research (and experience) is continuously uncovering exciting new management techniques. Unfortunately, not every physician specializes in diabetes or has the time to stay on top of it all—which may leave you a step behind.

The remainder of this book will focus on getting you up-to-date on the latest and greatest in diabetes treatment. That way, you can discuss your options openly and intelligently with your health-care team and decide what's truly in your best interests. In other words, instead of lagging behind, now is your chance to leap to the *forefront* of diabetes treatment!

Chapter Two

The Cornerstones of Diabetes Care

You would think that a book on "trends" in diabetes would focus solely on high-tech gadgets and the latest medications. Well, think again. The cornerstones of diabetes management (or "keystones," if you're a Pennsylvanian like me) remain our day-to-day lifestyle choices—particularly involving nutrition, physical activity, and emotional health. Research and experience are constantly teaching us better ways to utilize lifestyle tools to our fullest advantage.

WHAT'S NEW IN NUTRITION?

When it comes to managing diabetes, there are three things we need to think about when making food choices—calories, carbohydrates, and a little something called glycemic index.

Calories because we need to balance energy intake against energy expenditure.

Carbohydrates because they have the greatest immediate impact on blood sugar levels.

Glycemic Index because, in many cases, the rate at which food digests is just as important as *what* is being digested.

The Calorie Connection

Calories represent the energy content of food. Consume more energy than you burn, and the extra calories are typically stored in the form of fat. Consume less energy than you burn, and fat stores are broken down as a source of fuel. While achieving a healthy body weight is important for everyone, changes in weight—fat stores in particular—can have a major effect on the way insulin works.

When our body's fat cells grow, a few things change. Hormones are produced that cause insulin resistance throughout the body—particularly in muscle cells, which normally use more than 80 percent of the glucose taken into the body. When muscle cells become insulin resistant, additional insulin is required to control glucose levels. Also, with increasing fat stores and rising triglyceride levels in the blood, the liver begins to secrete extra glucose. Again, this causes an increase in insulin requirements.

The opposite occurs when we lose body fat. Suddenly, our muscles become more sensitive to insulin, and the liver eases up on its glucose secretion. The result, as you can imagine, is a decrease in insulin requirements.

One of the keys to managing diabetes over the long term is to achieve a healthy weight and stay there. Frequent swings in body size make diabetes very difficult to manage. Every time your fat stores increase or decrease, insulin dosage adjustments become necessary.

Since more people are interested in losing than gaining

weight, a few words about weight loss are in order. Because insulin ultimately dictates how much fuel our body's cells store, it will be necessary to reduce insulin doses in order to achieve safe, appropriate weight loss. This can be accomplished by cutting back on food intake, increasing physical activity, and lowering stress levels. Some diabetes medications can also help facilitate weight loss. These will be discussed later in this book.

Simply lowering insulin doses without making lifestyle changes (or adding certain medications) can produce dangerously high glucose levels. The term "diabulimic" has been used to describe those who intentionally under dose their insulin in order to run high blood sugar and lose weight (see Emotional Considerations at the end of this chapter). The problem with this practice, besides being very dangerous, is that high glucose often increases appetite and takes away energy, making it difficult to exercise. By contrast, making lifestyle changes without making appropriate insulin reductions can produce frequent hypoglycemia (low blood sugar), which will require extra food for treatment.

Glucose control is of primary importance when trying to lose weight. Elevated glucose levels drive hunger and sap energy, which makes it difficult to eat right and exercise. So, blood sugar management needs to take precedence.

In terms of weight-loss diets, here's some good news: It really doesn't matter which diet plan you choose. In comparing low-carb, low-fat, and overall reduced-calorie diets, the research has shown little difference in results. As long as the diet approach has you paying close attention to what you're eating, it will tend to work. However, diets that involve extreme restriction of any select nutrient, such as carbohydrates, can be very difficult to follow over the long term and may lead to nutrient deficiencies. Also, diet plans that involve ongoing social support systems seem to work better than those that have people doing it "on their own."

One other procedure that has shown promise in promoting weight loss and enhancing blood sugar control is "gastric banding." This is a surgical procedure that involves placing a band around the stomach so as to limit its ability to expand and empty normally. As the stomach fills up quickly, appetite becomes suppressed and food intake is reduced. However, as with any surgical procedure, there are potential complications and side effects, so discuss the details with your physician.

Count Your Carbs

Carbohydrates (or "carbs" for short) include simple sugars such as sucrose (table sugar), fructose (fruit sugar), lactose (milk sugar), and corn syrup, as well as complex carbohydrates, better known as "starch." Virtually all carbohydrates (except for fiber) are converted into glucose, which circulates through the bloodstream to nourish the body's cells. So, from a blood sugar control standpoint, it doesn't really matter if the carbs you eat are in the form of simple sugars or complex starches. Both will raise the blood sugar by the same amount. A cup of rice containing 40 grams of complex carbohydrate will raise the blood sugar just as much as a can of regular, sugar-sweetened soda that contains 40 grams of sugar. And both will do it pretty fast.

A key to successful blood sugar control is to know the amount of carb you are consuming, and match it to a corresponding dose of insulin. To match rapid-acting insulin to food, we use something called an "insulin-to-carb ratio." For example, a 1-to-10 (1:10) ratio means that one unit of insulin covers 10 grams of carbohydrate. A ratio of 1-to-20 (1:20) means that each unit covers 20 grams. If each unit covers 10g and you consume 65 grams, you will need 6.5 units of insulin (65 divided by 10 = 6.5).

The beauty of an I:C ratio is that it gives you the flexibility to eat as much or as little carbohydrate as you choose while still maintaining control of your blood sugars. *However, it remains important to space meals and snacks at least a few hours apart (three or more hours is optimal)* so that rapid-acting insulin can return the blood sugar to normal before you eat and raise it again. Even if carbs are counted carefully and appropriate doses of insulin are given, it is virtually impossible to control blood sugar when "grazing." Frequent munching puts you in a perpetual state of hyperglycemia, waiting for the insulin to kick in and bring the blood sugar back down to normal.

Incidentally, it is common to require different I:C ratios at different times of day. This is due to changes in hormone levels and physical activity (both of which affect insulin sensitivity). Many people find that they need their greatest insulin dose at breakfast and least in the middle of the day.

"Other" Dietary Influences

Carbs are not the only thing in our diets that can affect blood sugar levels. There are a few other factors to consider.

For many years, nutrition experts believed that dietary **protein** caused blood sugar to rise. Then, studies of mixed meals (meals containing carbs, protein, and fat) showed that protein had no effect. So what are we to believe?

As it turns out, the body uses protein for energy only when there are insufficient carbohydrates in the diet. When carbs are eaten, protein is used for purposes other than supplying blood sugar, such as bodily growth, cell and tissue repair, and creation of hormones and enzymes. But without carbs, protein becomes a source of glucose for nourishing the body's cells. For example, a breakfast consisting of eggs and sausage contains virtually no carbohydrates, but the blood sugar can rise anyway. When little or no carbohydrates are consumed, roughly 50 percent of protein is converted to glucose. This, of course, requires coverage with rapid-acting insulin.

Likewise, dietary fat's impact on blood sugar is usually of little significance. However, consumption of large amounts of fat can cause two distinct effects. First, it may slow the digestion of the carbohydrates that were consumed along with the fat, resulting in a more gradual post-meal glucose rise. Second, large amounts of dietary fat, particularly saturated fat, can produce their own delayed rise in the blood sugar level, related to a sharp increase in triglyceride levels in the bloodstream. For example, when having a high-fat dinner at a restaurant, the carbohydrates may take a few hours to "kick in" due to fat's slowing of digestion. Then, after you've gone to sleep, the blood sugar may rise again through the night as the liver begins secreting more glucose than usual (a result of high triglycerides in the bloodstream). This can usually be offset with extra basal/long-acting insulin after the meal.

Well-balanced meals with modest amounts of carbohydrate, protein, and fat are most likely to produce stable, predictable blood sugar levels—particularly when the carbohydrates are of a low-glycemic-index variety (see next section).

Alcoholic beverages have their own unique effect on blood sugar levels. Many drinks contain carbohydrates, which cause a short-term glucose rise. But alcohol has a tendency to lower blood sugar levels several hours later by keeping the liver from secreting its normal amount of glucose into the bloodstream. As a result, hypoglycemia can occur after drinking. When drinking, rapid insulin is usually needed right away to cover the carbohydrates. However, adjustments to long-acting/basal insulin may be needed to prevent a delayed blood sugar drop from the alcohol.

A natural stimulant, **caffeine** tends to cause a short-term rise in blood sugar levels. It does this by promoting the breakdown of fat (rather than sugar) for energy and stimulating the release of glucose by the liver. When consuming large amounts of caffeine, a small dose of rapid-acting insulin may be necessary.

Glycemic Index: It's All in the Timing

Glycemic index (GI) tells us how rapidly food raises the blood sugar level. Although virtually all carbohydrates convert into blood sugar eventually, some forms do so much faster than others. There are many books and web sites that have lists of glycemic index values for various foods, with scores ranging from 0 to 100 (with 100 being the fastest).[1] What the numbers represent is the percentage of carbohydrate that turns into blood glucose in the first two hours after the food is eaten. Foods with a high GI (greater than 70) tend

[1] *The Ultimate Guide to Accurate Carb Counting* by Gary Scheiner, 2007, Marlowe & Company, NY, NY.

to digest and convert to blood glucose the fastest, with a significant blood glucose "peak" occurring in 30 to 45 minutes. Foods with a moderate GI (45 to 70) digest a bit slower, resulting in a less pronounced blood glucose peak approximately one to two hours after they are consumed. Foods with a low GI (below 45) make a slow, gradual appearance in the bloodstream. The blood glucose peak is usually quite modest and may take several hours to occur.

Most starchy foods have a relatively high GI; they digest easily and convert into blood sugar quickly. Some starches, such as legumes (beans, nuts) and pasta digest quite slowly. Foods that have dextrose in them tend to have a very high GI. Table sugar (sucrose) has a moderate GI, while fructose (fruit sugar) and lactose (milk sugar) are somewhat slower at raising blood sugar. Foods that contain fiber or large amounts of fat tend to have lower GIs than comparable foods that do not.

For example, white bread has a glycemic index score of 71, while apples have a score of 38. This means that white bread will raise the blood sugar much faster than an apple. However, the total blood sugar rise from a slice of bread (containing 15g carb) and a small apple (containing 15g carb) will be the same ... the bread will just affect the blood sugar more quickly.

Why is glycemic index important? For those trying to control hunger and lose weight, low-glycemic-index foods tend to be more filling and create a sense of satiety. For those trying to minimize post-meal blood sugar spikes, low-GI foods are also beneficial in that they produce a more gradual rise in blood sugar.

For those who take rapid-acting insulin at mealtimes, the

glycemic index helps us to determine the optimal timing of the insulin. For foods with a high GI (greater than 70) it is usually best to take rapid insulin 20 to 30 minutes prior to eating. This will allow the insulin peak to coincide as closely as possible with the blood sugar peak, hence minimizing the post-meal spike. For foods with a moderate GI (approximately 45 to 69), it is usually best to take the insulin 5 to 10 minutes prior to eating. With low-GI foods (below 45), taking insulin prior to eating may cause the blood sugar to drop low and then rise high a few hours later as the food starts to take its effect. Taking insulin during or just after low-GI foods tends to work best.

High-GI Foods	Moderate-GI Foods	Low-GI Foods
Cereal	Pizza	Pasta
White Rice	Tacos	Beans and Nuts
White Potatoes	Juice	Berries
Most Salty Snacks	Brown Rice	Chocolate
Sugary Candies	Bananas	Milk

New Glucose Revolution Low GI Guide to Diabetes by Jennie Brand-Miller, J, 2006, Marlowe & Company, NY, NY.

What About Supplements?

If you're the type who thinks healthy nutrients come in pill form, think again. Both the American Diabetes Association and American Dietetic Association recommend that people at low risk for nutritional deficiencies (i.e., most people in industrialized countries) meet their nutritional needs with natural/ordinary food sources. However, those at risk for nutritional deficiencies (including those following very low-calorie diets, strict vegetarians, and the elderly) benefit from taking a daily multivitamin.

Some supplements, such as chromium and magnesium, have been thought to produce improvements in insulin sensitivity. However, most research studies have not supported this claim, particularly for those who already have healthy, well-balanced diets.

There are a few supplements and additives that have been shown to improve post-meal blood sugar control. These include fenugreek (seeds belonging to the same family as peanuts and chickpeas), ginseng (American or Asian), and vinegar.

Cinnamon (as a spice, not in pill form) has been linked to improved glucose control in people with type 2 diabetes. However, no studies have shown its effects in those with type 1. Recent studies have also shown beneficial effects from vitamin D supplementation for many people with diabetes, because it supports proper metabolism and immune system function. Given that many people with diabetes have a vitamin D deficiency, it may be worthwhile to have your level checked the next time you have lab work completed.

Some supplements have side effects, and most can be harmful when taken in very large doses. Speak to your physician or a qualified dietitian before starting to use any supplement.

LET'S GET PHYSICAL

We've known for many years that physical activity is a potent tool for lowering blood sugar. It does this by burning large amounts of glucose and improving the way insulin works—a process known as "insulin sensitization." Exercise makes the body's cells more efficient at using insulin to draw sugar out of the bloodstream. So what's new?

Muscle Up

Cardiovascular (aerobic) exercises, such as walking, swimming, and cycling, have always been considered beneficial for people with diabetes. Now, additional emphasis is being placed on muscle-building exercise. Strength-training, performed two or three times weekly in addition to cardiovascular exercise, can produce substantial improvements in insulin sensitivity and blood sugar control. Adding (or firming) muscle also raises the body's metabolic rate (calories burned at rest), which is helpful for those trying to lose weight or prevent unwanted weight gain.

Electronic Options

In many homes, "work"outs have been replaced by "play" outs. A number of companies produce video gaming systems with major physical activity components. These include Konami, which makes the Dance Dance Revolution (DDR) game for the Sony PlayStation; Nintendo, which makes WiiFit and Wii Conditioning games for the Wii system; SSD Company, which makes Xavix; Medway, which makes Cybex; and Light-Space Corp, which makes LightSpace games. These types of interactive games are becoming so popular that the term "exergaming" has been coined. Research has shown that many active video games burn as many calories as walking, jogging, and even running. Of course, there can be considerable differences based on the way you play the game. Nevertheless, there is something special about exergaming. People of all ages can have some serious fun while they get some serious exercise.

Offsetting Adrenaline

One of the most common struggles facing athletes with diabetes is the blood sugar rise that often accompanies an intense workout. Most commonly, blood sugar rises are seen during high-intensity, short-duration exercises and competitive sports. This is due primarily to adrenaline production, but it might also be related to rapid depletion of insulin or delayed digestion of food taken prior to the activity.

To prevent the blood sugar rise, many clinicians now advise taking a compensatory dose of rapid-acting insulin prior to certain activities. What's more, injecting the insulin into muscle (rather than fat) has been shown to hasten its action considerably. A conservative dose along with frequent blood glucose monitoring is recommended until you understand exactly how pre-workout insulin affects you specifically.

Delayed Onset Hypos

Another challenge often faced by people with diabetes is an unexpected drop in blood sugar several hours after certain types of workouts. Delayed blood sugar drops usually follow high-intensity, long-duration workouts. The timing of the drop varies from person to person and sport to sport. The causes include increased insulin sensitivity and the muscles' need to replenish their sugar stores (glycogen)following exhaustive exercise.

Once you have the ability to predict when a delayed drop will occur, prevention becomes relatively easy. Options include lowering basal/long-acting insulin post-exercise, reducing the dose of rapid-acting insulin at the next meal/snack, and consuming carbs (without taking rapid-acting insulin) several hours later.

Sensitivity in Reverse

From a blood sugar control standpoint, the emphasis has always been on dealing with the effects of increased physical activity. But what about the opposite? What happens when activity is much lower than usual?

Sitting (or lying) for long periods of time when you are usually up and moving tends to produce a gradual rise in the blood sugar level. Since your usual insulin doses are based on a standard level of physical activity, cutting back on that activity can result in less glucose - burning and a temporary decrease in insulin sensitivity.

Of course, it's easy to say, "Just don't be inactive for long periods of time." But reality sometimes gets in the way. There are long car trips, all-day meetings, football Sundays, and injuries that keep us from moving. Just as we usually have to decrease insulin when physical activity increases, we now know that insulin doses sometimes need to be increased for reductions in activity. Short-term inactivity (just a few hours) may simply require an increase in a mealtime insulin dose. Long-term inactivity may require increases in meal doses, correction doses (for elevated blood sugar), and basal insulin.

EMOTIONAL CONSIDERATIONS

The more we learn about how the mind influences health, the more we come to realize what we don't know. For instance, most people are unaware that the brain is a major consumer of glucose. Just as a computer heats up and uses more power when running multiple programs simultaneously, so does the brain during periods of multitasking, intense concentration, and sensory stimulation. That's why many people see a reduction in their blood sugar when they are doing things like studying, socializing, or even getting used to a new work or living environment.

Our emotions and mental state of mind have a tremendous impact on our ability to take care of diabetes, and some situations (such as those described above) have a direct effect on blood sugar levels. In fact, most major diabetes treatment centers now employ at least one mental health professional as part of their core team. Although a multitude of mental health conditions can impact diabetes, we're going to focus on three major problems—stress, depression, and eating disorders.

Stress and Glucose Control

Emotional stress (fear, anxiety, anger, excitement, tension) and physiological stress (illness, pain, infection, injury) cause the body to secrete stress hormones into the bloodstream. Chronic stress, such as job frustration or physical discomfort, causes an increase in cortisol levels throughout the day and night, which in turn elevates blood sugar on an ongoing basis. Sudden stress, such as getting into an accident or being threatened by an intruder, causes production of adrenal hormones. These cause the liver to secrete extra glucose and create a temporary state of insulin resistance (which, theoretically, ensures that there is extra glucose in the bloodstream to allow us to deal with the stressful situation).

For those without diabetes, stress-induced blood sugar rises are followed by an increase in insulin secretion, so the blood sugar rise is modest and momentary. For those with diabetes, stress can cause blood sugar to rise quickly or stay high on a long-term basis.

We all have some degree of stress in our lives. For some, severely stressful situations pop up frequently. And some find themselves in a constant stressful state. Some stress is healthy: it keeps us alert and helps us deal with crises. But excessive stress can cause a variety of physical and psychological symptoms. Physical symptoms include headaches, indigestion, stomach aches, sweaty palms, sleep difficulties, back pain, tight shoulders/neck, racing heart, and tiredness. Behavioral symptoms include excessive smoking or drinking, compulsive gum chewing, bossiness, being very critical of others, grinding one's teeth at night, and compulsive eating. Emotional symptoms include crying, nervousness, edginess, feeling powerless to change things, anger, loneliness, difficulty concentrating, forgetfulness, and loss of sense of humor.

Here are some effective ways to keep stress from impairing your diabetes control:

- Identify the people, things, and situations that cause stress for you. Being aware of your stressors allows you to prepare for them.
- Keep a sense of humor. Laughter is a tremendous outlet for stress.
- If waiting causes you stress, plan ahead with things to do while you wait.
- Find a temporary escape. Immerse yourself in music. Take

a vacation. Visit nature. Or just pamper yourself.

- Simplify your life and live within your means. Over-commitment is a major source of stress for many people.
- If you often feel overworked, prioritize and delegate. Learn how to say "no." No job is worth making yourself sick over.
- Find a release valve, also known as a catharsis. Some people benefit from writing down what is causing them stress and how it is making them feel. Others find comfort in talking things out with a friend.
- Exercise removes us from our problems. It improves blood flow to the brain so we can come up with creative solutions. It also makes us feel more in control of our bodies and our lives in general.
- Helping others and doing volunteer work can give your spirits a real lift. It's also a great way to refocus on things that really matter.
- Sleep deprivation can be a major source of physical and emotional stress. Invest in a comfortable bed and pillow. Avoid caffeine and heavy eating at night. Develop a bedtime "routine" that relaxes you and helps you to fall asleep. And allow yourself to get at least 6 to 8 hours of sleep nightly. If your partner has told you that you snore, or you awaken multiple times during the night (not related to your diabetes), talk to your doctor about whether you should be tested for sleep apnea.
- Meditation, accompanied by paced breathing, has the proven ability to calm and focus the mind, lower blood pressure, and put the body into a relaxed state. Practiced on a regular basis, meditation can be used to blunt

negative responses to stress.

- Practice progressive muscle relaxation. Tighten and release your muscles one group at a time, from face to toes, for about 10 seconds per muscle group. This forces your muscles to relax. Simply knowing how your muscles feel when relaxed will make it easier to tell when you're feeling tense in response to stress.

If you're not having much success on your own, consider seeking professional help. Most psychologists and psychiatrists are trained at helping their clients deal effectively with stress, sometimes through the use of medication.

Diabetes and Depression

Depression is a health disorder common among people with diabetes. Why? It's not known exactly, but people with diabetes are more likely than people without diabetes to develop depression. Several theories have been put forth as to why. In many cases, depression involves a chemical imbalance among neurotransmitters in the brain. Given that elevated glucose in the body's fluids and tissues presents a challenge to maintaining proper chemical balance, this may play a direct role. Increased stress has also been associated with depression. People with diabetes are prone to increased stress since we must manage a complicated condition in addition to taking care of everything else in our lives. Also, depression is often linked to a perceived loss of self-control. There are many aspects of blood sugar regulation that are beyond our control, such as environmental factors and the intricate balance of bodily hormones.

Those who suffer from diabetic complications (heart, nerve,

kidney, eye diseases) are particularly prone to depression. The more complications, the greater the risk. Research has shown that people with diabetes who have more than two complications have a 90 percent chance of also suffering from depression. A feeling of helplessness, which often occurs in people with multiple health problems, is thought to be the primary cause.

Whatever the mechanism, depression has serious implications for people with diabetes. Depression can lead to unhealthy meal patterns and excessive consumption of inappropriate foods. It often alters sleep patterns, resulting in excessive sleep, insomnia, or sleeping at odd times of day. And when sleep patterns change, so do daily hormone levels that influence glucose control. Sticking to an exercise program is also much more difficult when one is in a depressed state. And for that matter, just about every aspect of diabetes self-management (blood glucose monitoring, taking insulin, seeing health-care providers regularly) becomes more of a challenge.

Symptoms of depression include:
• Feeling sad often
• Crying spells
• Tiredness
• Dwelling on negative thoughts
• Dreading the future
• Contemplating suicide

The good news is that depression is treatable and manageable. Various forms of counseling with a qualified mental health counselor can work wonders. And modern types of antidepressant medications (SSRIs and SNRIs) can reverse depression symptoms with minimal side effects.

Talk to your physician if you are experiencing symptoms of depression. Like most illnesses, depression is not the fault of the person who experiences it, and it is not a sign of weakness. But if you are depressed and don't take action to treat it, you will seriously compromise your ability to control your diabetes.

Diabulimia

The two main eating disorders are anorexia nervosa and bulimia nervosa. People with anorexia restrict their food intake to stay or become thin. People with bulimia eat excessive amounts of food and then induce vomiting or take laxatives to purge the food from their body. A recent trend among young people with diabetes, particularly women who are dissatisfied with their body weight or shape, involves skipping or restricting insulin doses in order to lose weight. *Diabulimia*, as this is often called, can have devastating and permanent effects on the body.

Failure to take necessary doses of insulin causes blood sugar levels to rise very high and results in frequent urination, as the kidneys rid the body of the excess sugar in the bloodstream. This "purging" of the sugar from the body results in rapid weight loss and has been compared to the kind of purging done by those with bulimia. Skipping insulin doses to lose weight puts an individual at risk for serious short-term health problems, including dehydration, fatigue, infection, ketoacidosis, and loss of muscle tissue. Individuals who engage in this practice are also at a very high risk for developing blindness, kidney disease, heart disease, and nerve disorders at an early age. Another very serious complication of these disorders is electrolyte imbalance, which can cause heart attacks even in people who are quite young.

Although the risks associated with restricting or omitting insulin are severe, the most alarming aspect of this behavior is how widespread it has become. Studies have shown that young women with diabetes are more than twice as likely to develop an eating disorder compared to those without diabetes. And one study found that nearly one out of three adolescent women with type 1 diabetes have skipped or restricted insulin doses in order to lose weight.

While diabetes itself does not cause eating disorders, it can set the stage. Those with insulin-dependent diabetes must pay close attention to their diet and exercise, constantly monitoring their blood sugar levels and carbohydrate intake. This near-obsessive relationship with food can increase the risk of eating disorders in some individuals, particularly young girls.

Warning signs of an eating disorder include:

- changes in eating habits (eating more but still losing weight)
- unexplained weight loss
- unexplained hyperglycemia (high blood sugar)
- repeated bouts of severe low blood sugar
- extremely high A1c results
- frequent hospitalizations for poor blood sugar control
- low energy levels
- frequent urination

- frequent infections
- anxiety about or avoidance of being weighed
- switching of meal-planning approaches
- delay in puberty, irregular or no menses
- exercising more than necessary to stay fit

Treatment requires a collaborative effort between an eating disorder/mental health specialist and a diabetes management team. In some cases, medication may be used to alleviate depression and anxiety symptoms. Preventive efforts should focus on developing a healthy relationship with food and insulin. This includes establishing a balanced, flexible approach to eating in terms of food types and times.

The key to dealing with an eating disorder, as was the case with depression, is recognition of the symptoms, acceptance that it is a health condition that requires treatment, and seeking out appropriate treatment. Eating disorders can be treated, and people do recover from them, but the longer symptoms are ignored, the harder it is to turn them around and deal with the harsh effects they have had on the body.

Chapter Three

Medication
Innovations

At last check, there were nine different classes of medications for treating diabetes, each working on different parts of the body in their own unique ways. There are also a multitude of brands within each class. As if that wasn't complicated enough, there are also combination medications that mix multiple prescriptions in one pill.

If you're lucky enough to see a board-certified endocrinologist who specializes in diabetes, you should receive reasonably sound advice when it comes to choosing the right medications and setting the right doses. If not (and at least 90 percent of people with diabetes do not), you're probably working with someone who deals with literally hundreds of health conditions, each with its own long list of treatment options. As you can imagine, they are not likely to be up to speed on the latest diabetes medications and insulin programs.

Regardless of the expertise of your medical provider, it is to your advantage to know as much as possible about all of the medical options for treating diabetes. After all, it's your body, and nobody knows your situation better than you.

And nobody stands to benefit more from proper care and treatment than you.

MODERN INSULIN THERAPY

Before jumping into a huge pile of pills, let's focus on the most powerful and natural form of diabetes treatment—insulin therapy. Whether your body still produces its own insulin or you take it via injection, the key to successful blood sugar control is to match the insulin you receive to the insulin your body needs.

To understand the body's insulin needs, we need to consider the two "Bs"—"basal" or "background" insulin, along with "boluses" or "bunches" of insulin.

Basal Basics

Basal insulin's job is to take the glucose secreted by the liver and pack it into the body's cells to burn for fuel. One of the liver's most important functions is to store glucose (in a dense form called "glycogen") and secrete it steadily into the blood-stream. This provides the body's vital organs with a constant source of fuel. A healthy pancreas produces a small amount of insulin all day and all night to match the liver's glucose production. Not only does this ensure a steady supply of energy for the body's cells, it also keeps the liver from dumping out too much glucose all at once. Too little basal insulin, or a complete lack of insulin, would result in a sharp rise in blood sugar levels.

So, you might say that basal insulin and the liver are in balance with each other. Too much basal insulin will cause the blood sugar to drop between meals and overnight. Too little basal insulin and the blood sugar would be rising continuously. Each person's basal insulin requirements are unique. Typically, basal insulin needs are highest during the night and early morning, and lowest in the middle of the day. This is due to the production of blood sugar–raising hormones during the night and enhanced sensitivity to insulin that comes with daytime physical activity.

Figure 1 shows typical basal insulin requirements for people with insulin-dependent diabetes by age group. For those with type 2 diabetes, basal insulin requirements tend to be "flatter" (lacking in peaks and valleys) since the pancreas still produces some insulin on its own.

During a person's growth years (prior to age 21), basal insulin tends to be relatively high throughout the night, drop through the morning hours, and gradually increase from noon to midnight. Most adults (age 21+) exhibit a "peak" in basal insulin requirements during the early morning hours. This is commonly referred to as a "dawn phenomenon."

Basal insulin can be supplied in a variety of ways. Intermediate-acting insulin (NPH or isophane) taken once daily will

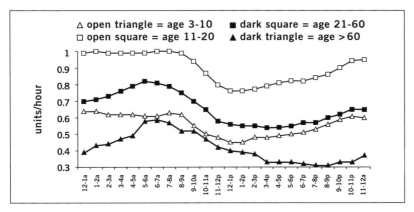

Figure 1: Typical basal insulin requirements by age.

✳ Trend

Peakless, long-acting insulin has replaced NPH as the basal insulin of choice.

usually provide background insulin around the clock, albeit at much higher levels 4 to 8 hours after injection and at much lower levels 12 to 24 hours after injection. Long-acting basal insulins (degludec, glargine, and detemir) offer relatively peakless insulin levels around the clock. Insulin pumps deliver rapid-acting insulin in small pulses throughout the day and night. With a pump, tiny pulses of rapid-acting insulin are delivered every couple of minutes to produce a constant low level of insulin in the bloodstream. The basal insulin level can be increased at certain hours of the day and decreased at others in order to match the body's varying basal insulin needs. It is also possible to combine various forms of long-acting insulin to simulate the body's normal basal insulin secretion.

Summary of Available Basal Insulin Options

	Action Profile	Advantages	Disadvantages
NPH Isophane (also called "intermediate-acting" insulin)	Begins working: 1-2 hours Peaks: 4-8 hours Lasts: 12-18 hours	Pronounced peak to offset "dawn phenomenon" Can be mixed in one syringe (or pen) with rapid-acting insulin Relatively inexpensive	Two or more injections daily required for 24-hour basal coverage Unpredictable; action (onset, peak, duration) can vary considerably from day to day Must maintain a consistent meal schedule to prevent hypoglycemia Must be rolled/mixed prior to injection

	Action Profile	Advantages	Disadvantages
Tresiba (degludec)	Begins working: 1-2 hours Peaks: no peaks Lasts: 2-3 days	Timing of injections may vary Very stable/consistent action	When starting takes several days to ramp up to stable level in bloodstream No "peak" to offset dawn phenomenon
Glargine (Lantus)	Begins working: 1-2 hours Peaks: no peaks Lasts: 20-24 hours	One injection/day usually provides 24-hour coverage Low risk of hypoglycemia due to lack of a peak Allows some flexibility with meal and sleep times	No "peak" to offset dawn phenomenon Cannot mix with rapid insulin in same syringe/pen Relatively expensive
Detemir (Levemir)	Begins working: 1-2 hours Peaks: mildly at 6-12 hours Lasts: 16-24 hours	Low risk of hypogycemia due to limited "peak" Very consistent action profile regardless of dosage amount Allows some flexibility with meal and sleep times	Usually requires two injections daily to provide 24-hour coverage Cannot mix with rapid insulin in the same syringe/pen Relatively expensive
Insulin Pump	Micro-pulses of rapid insulin every few minutes. Continuous action, peaks at the time of day set by the user.	Can vary basal insulin level hourly to match body's precise needs Temporary/short-term adjustments can be made for lifestyle activities Can deliver in very small and precise increments Unlimited schedule flexibility	Lack of long-acting insulin means that ketoacidosis DKA can develop if insulin delivery is stopped for several hours Must stay connected to the pump almost continuously

For those who don't mind a bit of creativity, some patients and clinicians have begun using combinations of basal insulin therapies. For those on injection ther-

apy who experience an overnight or early-morning blood sugar rise, a combination of degludec, glargine, or detemir (taken once daily in the morning) and NPH (taken near bedtime) can provide basal insulin coverage that mimics the body's normal basal production. For those who use insulin pumps and must disconnect for extended periods of time or are susceptible to ketoacidosis, it is feasible to take a low dose of glargine or detemir in the morning, overlapped with the pump's basal insulin delivery. Of course, the pump's basal rates would need to be reduced throughout the day and night to compensate for the presence of long-acting insulin.

Bolus Insulin

In addition to basal insulin, fast-acting insulin is necessary to offset the rapid blood sugar rise that occurs after eating carbohydrates (sugars and starches). Carbohydrates usually take 10 to 20 minutes to begin raising the blood sugar, with a high point occurring 30 to 90 minutes following a meal or snack. Bolus insulin is also used to bring high blood sugars down to normal.

Not everyone who takes insulin requires fast-acting insulin at mealtimes, but most do. In some cases, people with type 2 diabetes can still produce enough of their own insulin after meals to minimize post-meal blood sugar spikes. However, many people with type 2 diabetes, and everyone with type 1, require bolus insulin at mealtimes.

Prior to 1999, the only bolus insulin available was called "regular" insulin. It came under different names based on the company that made it, such as Novolin R (from Novo Nordisk) and Humulin R (from Lilly), the R in the name standing for regular. One of the major problems with regular insulin is that it works too slowly to cover most foods. Its action also varies considerably depending on where it is injected into the body.

Today, we have "rapid-acting insulin analogs" that work much faster and are more consistent and predictable than regular. These include lispro (brand name Humalog), aspart (brand names NovoLog and NovoRapid), and glulisine (brand name Apidra). Because they work faster, rapid-acting analogs bring high blood sugars down more quickly (so you spend less time above target), and reduce the blood sugar "spike" that occurs after meals and snacks. Whereas regular insulin must be taken 30 minutes or more before meals in order to have a chance at managing the post-meal blood sugar peak, rapid analogs can usually be taken just a few minutes before eating.

What exactly are "analogs"? They are actually regular insulin molecules whose chemical structure has been altered slightly. After injection, regular insulin molecules tend to stick to each other under the skin, and this slows down the rate at which they absorb and act. Unit for unit, rapid-acting analogs work just as hard as regular, but the slight change in their structure keeps them from sticking together. This allows for much quicker action.

One other bolus insulin option is U-500 regular. U-500 is five times more concentrated and powerful than ordinary U-100 regular insulin, but its action is quite a bit slower. In fact, the action profile of U-500 resembles that of NPH, one of the intermediate-acting basal insulins. For this reason, U-500 use is limited to those with extreme insulin resistance who require several hundred units of insulin per day. An amount this large can be impractical to administer via injections or a pump, so much smaller doses of U-500 can be used.

Currently Available Bolus Insulin Options

	Action Profile	Advantages	Disadvantages
Lispro (Humalog) **Aspart (NovoLog, NovoRapid)** **Glulisine (Apidra)**	Begins working: 10-20 minutes Peaks: 1-2 hours Lasts: 1-5 hours	May be taken shortly before meals Reduction in post-meal blood sugar spikes Brings elevated blood sugar down relatively quickly Consistent action profile regardless of injection site Blood sugar should stabilize 3-5 hours after injecting	Relatively expensive Quicker onset of DKA with pump malfunction
Regular (Humulin, Novolin	Begins working: 20-30 minutes Peaks: 2-4 hours Lasts: 6-8 hours	Relatively inexpensive Slower onset of DKA with pump malfunction	Must be taken well in advance of meals (30 minutes or more) Significant post-meal blood sugar spikes are common Takes many hours to bring high blood sugar down to normal Action profile can vary based on site of injection Blood sugar may drop quickly 3-5 hours after injection
U-500 Regular	Starts: 1-3 hours Peaks: 3-8 hours Lasts: 8-12 hours	Allows smaller volume dosing for those with very high insulin requirements	Slow, broad peak results in high blood sugar peaks after meals Takes many hours to lower high blood sugar

Although rapid-acting insulin analogs are generally considered superior to regular as a bolus insulin, there are situations where regular insulin may be preferred. For example, when consuming slowly digested foods (such as pasta, beans, dairy products, or very-high-fat meals), rapid-acting insulin may actually work too quickly. This can cause low blood sugar soon after eating, followed by a gradual rise over the next several hours. Regular insulin may be a better option with these types of foods.

> ## ❊ Trend
>
> *Insulin "cocktails" consisting of various types of bolus insulin can be used to cover mixed meals.*

Some people find that combining regular insulin with a rapid analog can work well with mixed meals that contain some slowly digesting and some rapidly digesting carbohydrates. For example, a meal consisting of bread (which raises blood sugar rapidly) and pasta (which acts slowly) can be covered with a bolus consisting of half regular insulin and half rapid insulin mixed in the same syringe.

Individuals with gastroparesis may also benefit from using regular (or a regular/rapid mix) at mealtimes. Gastroparesis slows the rate at which food digests and often requires a bolus that acts more gradually than the usual rapid analogs.

Finally, for those who are very sensitive to small doses of insulin and do not have access to an insulin pump (which permits dosing in very small increments), it is possible to dilute lispro (Humalog) rapid-acting insulin to a concentration as low as 10 percent. This permits dosing in tenths or twentieths of a unit (using syringes with ½-unit markings).

The process for diluting insulin requires several steps and must be performed in a sterile

✳ Trend

For those on injections who are very sensitive to insulin, diluting the insulin can allow dosing in tenths or twentieths of a unit.

manner, so don't hesitate to ask for the assistance of your local pharmacist. Equipment required includes:

- A fresh vial of lispro (Humalog) insulin
- A vial of sterile diluent, obtained by your pharmacist from Lilly Corp.
- A new 100 unit (1cc) insulin syringe

The steps for diluting the insulin to 10 percent of its normal concentration (also called U-10) are as follows:

- Inject 100 units of air into the diluent vial.
- Withdraw 100 units of diluent into the syringe and discard (spray into trash).
- Inject 100 units of air into the Humalog insulin vial.
- Withdraw 100 units Humalog insulin into the syringe.
- Inject insulin into the diluent vial.
- Roll the vial between hands to mix.

This gives you a vial containing 1000 units of Humalog that has been diluted to 10 percent of its usual concentration. The diluted insulin is good for one month and is stable at room temperature, but it should be rolled in the hands to ensure an even mixture before each use. Don't forget that each unit of this mixture only contains one-tenth of a unit of actual insulin! The chart below can help you convert your usual doses to 10 percent diluted doses.

Units of U-10	Units of Insulin	Units of U-10	Units of Insulin	Units of U-10	Units of Insulin
1	.1	11	1.1	21	2.1
2	.2	12	1.2	22	2.2
3	.3	13	1.3	23	2.3
4	.4	14	1.4	24	2.4
5	.5	15	1.5	25	2.5
6	.6	16	1.6	26	2.6
7	.7	17	1.7	27	2.7
8	.8	18	1.8	28	2.8
9	.9	19	1.9	29	2.9
10	1.0	20	2.0	20	3.0

Combining Basal and Bolus

Selecting the best insulin program to meet your needs depends on a number of factors. If you have type 2 diabetes, latent autoimmune diabetes of adulthood (LADA), or are in the honeymoon phase of type 1 diabetes, your pancreas may produce sufficient amounts of insulin to meet some of your insulin requirements. Your physician can perform blood tests to determine if this is the case. If so, you may be able to get by with just a daily injection of basal insulin or an occasional shot of bolus insulin to offset a particular incident of high blood sugar or a particularly large meal.

Otherwise, it is best to utilize a program that combines both basal and bolus insulin. A number of options are available, so let's take a look at the features, advantages, and disadvantages of each.

Pre-Mixed Insulin (70/30 or 75/25) Taken Twice Daily

Pre-mixed includes both intermediate-acting insulin (NPH) and a rapid-acting analog in the same vial or pen. The larger number (70 or 75) represents the percentage that is NPH.

One of the premixed formulation's major shortcomings is that you cannot change the proportion of NPH to rapid insulin. If you need more rapid insulin, you must also take more intermediate (NPH) insulin, and vice versa. With the morning NPH insulin peaking in the afternoon, meals and snacks must be consumed at specific times and in specific amounts. Changes to the usual schedule can lead to high and low glucose levels. Exercise during the day can also produce lows with this type of insulin schedule unless extra carbohydrates are consumed. The evening NPH insulin peaks around midnight and dissipates as dawn approaches, predisposing most users to low blood sugar in the middle of the night and highs at wake-up.

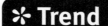

✳ Trend

Premixed insulin is generally considered inferior for those using a basal/bolus approach.

Perhaps the only advantage to this program is the ease of administration. Only two injections per day are required, and premixed formulations eliminate the possibility of accidentally mixing up insulin types.

Morning NPH and Rapid, Dinner Rapid, Bedtime NPH

The morning dose of NPH and rapid insulin is mixed manually by the user in one syringe, so the dose of rapid insulin can be adjusted based on the amount of carbohydrates consumed. Likewise, rapid insulin at dinner is not part of a premixed formulation and can be adjusted as needed. By taking the evening NPH at bedtime instead of dinner, the peak is shifted to early morning (around the time of the dawn phenomenon), thus improving the chances for stable glucose levels during the night.

There are still many disadvantages to this program. Midmorning, midday, and afternoon food intake and physical activity must be structured and monitored carefully. There is little schedule flexibility. And you still have morning and evening injections of NPH that must be taken on schedule, but the action profiles of these injections may vary from day to day.

Bedtime NPH with Rapid Insulin at Each Meal

This, along with all of the following programs, falls under the heading of "multiple daily injection" (MDI) therapy. People used to go to great lengths to avoid taking more shots. But then, reality set in. With the miniscule, virtually painless pen needles and syringe needles we have today, most people have come to realize that the injections are the easiest thing about living with diabetes. It's the challenging lifestyle and uncontrolled blood sugars that can be tough to live with.

With this type of MDI program, NPH insulin taken at bedtime provides an early-morning peak to cover the dawn phenomenon, as well as a prolonged "tail" of action that ensures the presence of at least some basal insulin throughout the day. However, the peak and duration of NPH can vary from day to day, and the tapering action of the insulin in the afternoon and evening may result in a blood sugar rise late in the day.

This type of plan requires an injection of rapid-acting insulin at every meal and snack, although snacks that are very low in carbohydrates may not require an injection. Many people find that insulin pens make frequent injections less of a chore. Pens that deliver in half-unit increments are available for those who are sensitive to small insulin doses. For those who want to avoid frequent needle sticks, injection ports can be used (see details in Delivery Options).

✳ Trend

MDI (multiple daily injections) and pump therapy are considered the optimal approaches to diabetes care.

Taking rapid-acting insulin with each meal and snack gives you the freedom to eat what you choose, since the dose can be matched to the amount of carbohydrate being eaten. This process also allows adjustments for variations in physical activity, as well as timely corrections for glucose readings that are above target.

Long-Acting Basal Insulin (glargine or detemir) with Rapid-Acting Insulin at Each Meal

Degludec (Tresiba) or glargine (Lantus) taken once daily in the morning or evening, or detemir (Levemir) taken twice daily, provides a steady level of basal insulin for about 24 hours.

Use of long-acting basal insulin has its pros and cons. The consistent absorption and lack of a significant "peak" minimize the risk of hypoglycemia. However, glucose levels may drop gradually between meals during the daytime hours since basal insulin needs tend to be lower then. There may also be a rise overnight or in the early morning hours when basal insulin needs tend to be higher.

Injections of rapid-acting insulin are necessary with every meal and snack. And unlike NPH, which can be mixed in the same syringe with rapid-acting insulin, glargine and detemir must be injected separately from rapid insulin.

Morning Basal Insulin with Bedtime NPH and Rapid Insulin at Each Meal

A low dose of injected basal insulin (degludec, glargine, or levemir) in the morning maintains relatively steady glucose levels between meals during the day, and a nighttime dose of NPH offsets the dawn phenomenon in the middle of the night and early morning. The dose of NPH can be adjusted based on factors that might influence overnight glucose levels, such as illness, heavy exercise during the day, and high-fat meals late in the day. As with any MDI program, injections of rapid-acting insulin are necessary with every meal and snack.

Insulin Pump Therapy

Insulin pumps combine the best of both basal and bolus delivery options. Pumps hold only rapid-acting insulin, but deliver tiny pulses every few minutes to provide a continuous flow of basal insulin. The pump is unique in that it allows the level of basal insulin to vary based on the time of day. For example, the basal program below, which repeats automatically every 24 hours, provides a higher rate of basal insulin in the middle of the night and predawn hours and a lower rate in the morning and afternoon.

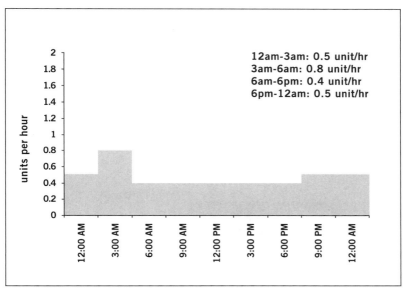

units per hour

12am-3am: 0.5 unit/hr
3am-6am: 0.8 unit/hr
6am-6pm: 0.4 unit/hr
6pm-12am: 0.5 unit/hr

Sample Basal Program on an Insulin Pump

At meal and snack times, the pump user programs a bolus of insulin to cover dietary carbohydrates or bring a high blood sugar down toward normal. Modern pumps have built-in bolus calculators. The user simply enters their blood sugar and grams of carb, and the pump calculates a suggested bolus amount.

There are other unique advantages as well as drawbacks to using an insulin pump. These are described in the following section.

INSULIN DELIVERY OPTIONS

Disposable syringes are the traditional method for delivering insulin. When choosing insulin syringes, select the smallest size possible given your usual dose. This allows for the greatest dosage accuracy. Low-dose syringes are now available that have ½-unit markings. If you rarely require more than 20 units in a single injection, choose 0.3 cc (30-unit) syringes with ½-unit markings. If you sometimes require more than 20 units but rarely take more than 40 units in a single injection, choose 0.5 cc (50-unit) syringes. If you often require more than 40 units in a single injection, choose 1 cc (100-unit) syringes.

As far as the syringe needle, thinner is always better. "Thinness" is measured by gauge. The higher the gauge, the thinner the needle. Make sure your syringe needles are at least 30 gauge. Depending on your pharmacy or supplier, you may be able to get syringes with needles that are as thin as 31 or 32 gauge.

> **✻ Trend**
>
> *Unless you take very large doses of insulin, short pen and syringe needles should work fine.*

The optimal needle length depends on your body type, although needles longer than 8 mm are rarely necessary, even if you are very heavy. Using needles that are too thick or too long can cause unnecessary pain and bruising and may result in accidental injection into muscle rather than fat. However, when large doses (greater than 50 units) are required, longer needles may be preferred to prevent leakage at the injection site.

Insulin syringes are produced by the following companies:

- Abbott (Precision Sure-Dose)
  800-252-6782; www.abbottdiabetescare.com

- Allison Medical (SureComfort)
  800-886-1618; www.allisonmedical.com
- Becton Dickinson / BD (UltraFine)
  888-232-2737; www.bddiabetes.com
- Perrigo Diabetes Care (Monoject, ReliOn)
  800-461-7448; www.canamcare.com

For those looking for a safe, fast, accurate, convenient, and discreet alternative to syringes, **insulin pens** are the answer. Pens cut down substantially on medical waste—something that has made them the standard for giving insulin in most countries outside the United States. Using a pen is as simple as turning a dial to the desired dose, inserting the small disposable needle into the skin, and pressing a button to deliver the insulin. In addition to visualizing the dose in the pen's display window, the user can hear and feel "clicks" as the dial is turned.

Pens either come prefilled or with disposable insulin cartridges. The disposable needles used on insulin pens are thinner and sharper than traditional syringe needles, and hence more comfortable. Select a pen needle length that is appropriate for your body type. Four to eight millimeter needles suit most people. Prefilled pens containing 300 units of long-acting/basal insulin (glargine, detemir, or premixed insulin) or rapid-acting insulin (aspart, lispro, glulisine) deliver in whole-unit increments. Durable pens that

✳ Trend

Insulin pens are superior to syringes in just about every way.

take 300-unit disposable cartridges of rapid-acting insulin can dose in either whole or half-unit increments. If you are fairly sensitive to insulin, consider using a pen that delivers in half-units.

If you often require doses of one unit or less, a pen may not be your best option, as dosing accuracy is not as precise as syringes at very low insulin doses. With any type of insulin pen, the pen needle must be kept in the skin for 5 to 10 seconds following the injection to ensure complete insulin delivery.

Insulin pens are available from all insulin manufacturers. Some medical device companies also produce pens that use disposable insulin cartridges:

- Eli Lilly (KwikPen, Luxura HD, Memoir)
  800-545-5979; www.lillydiabetes.com
- Novo Nordisk (FlexPen, NovoPen 3, NovoPen Junior)
  800-727-6500; www.novonordisk-us.com
- Owen Mumford (Autopen Classic)
  (U.K.) 01993 812021;
  www.owenmumford.com/en/range/6/autopen
- Sanofi-Aventis (SoloSTAR)
  800-981-2491; www.lantus.com/; www.apidra.com

Pen needles may be obtained from the following:
- Becton Dickinson / BD (Ultra-Fine, Nano)
  888-232-2737; www.bddiabetes.com
- Perrigo (Clickfine)
  800-461-7448; www.canamcare.com
- Novo Nordisk (NovoFine)
  800-727-6500;
  www.novolog.com/devices-alt_devices.asp

- Owen Mumford (Unifine)
  (U.K.) 01993 812021;
  www.owenmumford.com/us/range/30/unifine-pentips

Injection ports are an option for those with a significant dread of frequent needle sticks. These devices require just one needle stick every two or three days in order to place a tiny plastic infusion tube below the skin. Injections are given into a port that sits on the skin surface, so there is no skin puncture or discomfort whatsoever when insulin is injected into the port. The port must be changed every 2 to 3 days and should only be used for one insulin type (i.e., bolus doses).

Two types of injection ports are available. The i-port (Patton Medical, 877-763-7678, www.i-port.com) inserts at a 90-degree angle to the skin and comes with its own spring-loaded insertion device. The Insuflon (Unomedical in Denmark, 011 45 4816 7000, www.infusion-set.com) inserts at a 30-degree angle to the skin and must be inserted manually.

Insulin pumps are beeper-sized, battery-operated devices that infuse rapid-acting insulin into the body. Pumps are programmed by the user to deliver tiny pulses of rapid-acting insulin every few minutes throughout the day and night (basal insulin), and larger doses at mealtimes (bolus insulin). The insulin is delivered by way of a small, flexible plastic tube or a tiny needle that is placed just below the skin. The infusion set, as this is called, must be changed every couple of days in order to prevent clogging and infection and ensure consistent insulin absorption. Recent research and consensus papers have pointed to the value of frequent infusion device changes (every 48 hours) in order to prevent elevated blood sugar levels and the development of a chronic skin problem called lipodystrophy— damage to the fat layer below the skin caused by recurrent infusion of insulin in the same localized area. When the fat is damaged, insulin does not absorb properly.

Most infusion devices, including those that insert at a 30- to 45-degree angle, can be inserted automatically using a spring-loaded device; others are inserted by hand. The infusion device is usually worn on the abdomen, buttocks, or hip. It is taped in place securely, so it is not likely to "pull out" while you sleep or exercise. Infusion devices feature a disconnect mechanism that allows you to temporarily unhook the pump and tubing for situations such as bathing, contact sports, and intimacy. The tube that connects the pump to the infusion device is very strong and comes in different lengths. Some of the newer pumps are referred to as "patch" pumps —the pump itself sticks directly to the skin and has its own built-in tube that infuses the insulin below the skin. Patch pumps are programmed via a remote control device.

Modern pumps feature built-in bolus calculators. Buttons are used to enter specific blood sugar levels and carbohydrate amounts, and the pump calculates a recommended dose based on the formulas programmed by you and your health-care team. Pumps can even deduct previous bolus insulin that is still working in your body so you don't accidentally overdose. The bolus doses are very precise, with increments as low as one-fortieth of a unit. All pumps offer the option of delivering mealtime boluses all at once or over an extended period of time—in case you expect your meal to take a while to digest. And each pump keeps a record of all this information in its memory for on-screen recall or downloading to a computer.

As mentioned previously, one very unique aspect of pump therapy is the ability to fine-tune and adjust basal insulin levels during different phases of the day and night. By matching basal insulin to the liver's normal output of glucose, blood sugars should hold steady between meals and during the night. This allows you to vary your schedule as much as you like in terms of meals, activities, sleep, and travel. Basal insulin levels can also be adjusted on-the-fly for circumstances such as menstrual cycles, pregnancy, stress, illness, high-fat meals, and extended exercise.

Benefits of pump therapy include:

- **Better Blood Sugars** Pump users tend to have lower A1cs and less glucose variability than those on injections.
- **Fewer Lows** This is mainly due to the replacement of basal insulin with predictable (and adjustable) basal delivery from the pump that, when set correctly, should hold glucose levels steady between meals and overnight.
- **A More Flexible Lifestyle** Due to between-meal glucose stability, the pump lets you choose your own schedule as far as eating, sleeping, and exercising.
- **Bolus Calculations** Raise your hand if you enjoy doing math. Modern pumps calculate your bolus doses for you

based on your blood sugar, carbohydrate, and insulin "on board" from previous boluses.

- **Precise Dosing** Pumps deliver insulin to the nearest tenth, twentieth, or fortieth of a unit, depending on the model.
- **Convenience** There is no need to draw up syringes and give an injection every time you need insulin; just reach for your pump and press a few buttons.
- **No Shots** Multiple daily insulin injections can be uncomfortable and may cause skin trauma. Pumps only require a needle stick once every 2 to 3 days to replace the infusion device.
- **Easy Adjustments for Real Life** Temporary basal insulin changes help maintain stable blood sugar during periods of growth, illness, seasonal sports, dining out, and menstruation. The ability to deliver boluses all at once or over a prolonged period of time can be helpful when dining out or having holiday meals.
- **Weight Control** Pumps allow you to eat what and when you choose; no snacking required.
- **Data Analysis** Insulin pumps store a great deal of historical information that can be displayed on-screen or transmitted to computer programs for analysis and fine-tuning.

Potential drawbacks to pump therapy include:
- **Cost** Although most insurance plans cover insulin pumps and supplies, there are often co-pays and deductibles that must be met.
- **A Learning Curve** Don't expect good control right away. It usually takes a month or two to determine the right

basal and bolus doses and to adjust to using the pump correctly.

- **Inconvenience** Wearing the pump virtually all the time can be awkward once in a while.
- **Technical Difficulties** Pumps are generally quite durable, but they are prone to occasional tubing clogs, electronic/ software glitches, and damage due to wear and tear.
- **Skin Problems** Skin can become irritated from infusion set adhesive, and infections can occur if infusion sets are worn too long or inserted improperly. Insulin absorption can be hindered if infusion sets are not changed regularly and sites are not rotated properly.
- **Ketosis** The absence of long-acting insulin with pump use can present a problem if insulin delivery is interrupted for more than a few hours. Blood sugar can rise very quickly, and ketones (acids that result from breaking down too much fat and not enough sugar for energy) may appear if the problem is not corrected in a timely manner.
- **Infusion Set Changes** Every couple of days, the pump user must change his/her infusion device. This 3 to 10 minute procedure involves numerous steps and can be uncomfortable or traumatic for the novice pump user.

It is important to note that insulin pumps do not control blood sugars automatically. Hopefully, in a future edition of this book, this will be the case. But at this point, it takes a skilled, educated, and motivated user to operate the pump properly and benefit to the fullest.

In recent years, the major advances in pump therapy have focused on both clinical and cosmetic aspects. Clinically, the inclusion of "insulin on board" (IOB) or "active insulin" in bolus calculations has made pumping much safer and more effective than ever before. IOB represents the amount of insulin still believed to be working in the body from boluses given during the past several hours. By deducting IOB from certain types of boluses, it is safe to correct elevated glucose readings at any time—even shortly after a meal.

Another clinically beneficial improvement involves the use of finer increments in setting basal rates and insulin-to-carb ratios. Those

✳ Trend

All basal/bolus insulin users should make adjustments for "Insulin On Board." Modern pumps do this automatically.

who are very sensitive to small doses of insulin will be pleased to know that basal rates on most pumps can now be set in increments of 0.025 units per hour. This is important because very small basal changes can have significant effects on those who are on low doses of insulin. Those who require large doses at mealtimes will benefit from the fact that many pumps now allow setting insulin-to-carb (I:C) ratios in tenths of a gram (for example, 1 unit for every 3.3 grams of carbohydrate). This is important because changing I:C ratios in whole-number intervals, such as from 1:5 to 1:4, or from 1:2 to 1:3, results in a huge change in the bolus amount. Adding the decimal allows safer and more gradual fine-tuning.

Increasingly, the need to adjust insulin for variations in physical activity is taking center stage. For the first time, a pump system (the Accu-Chek Combo) incorporates a bolus multiplier into the bolus calculations. Essentially, once a bolus is calculated, it can be tagged with a "health event" that adjusts the bolus upward or downward by a pre-programmed percentage. Thus, boluses can easily be adjusted for increases or decreases in physical activity.

One other clinically beneficial change involves the inclusion of missed bolus reminders. Many pumps now allow the user to set time intervals (such as 6AM to 9AM) during which a bolus is expected to be taken. If no bolus is delivered by the end of this time interval, the user is alerted. This is important because most pump users forget to bolus for their meals once in a while, and missing boluses can have a major impact on both short-term control and the A1c level.

Improvements have also been made in pump data collection and analysis. These will be discussed later in this book.

Cosmetically (and conveniently) speaking, pumps are becoming smaller and less obtrusive. "Patch" pumps are easier to conceal than traditional pumps. Assorted colors and customized covers/stickers are being made available. Stronger, sleeker clips have been designed. And many pumps (including Animas, Insulet, and Tandem) have moved from traditional black-on-olive LCD screens to bright, full-color displays. One recently approved pump (Tandem), as well as several that are in the research and development pipeline, has incorporated the power of touch-screen technology. In addition, most pumps link with a blood glucose meter to make bolus calculations easier and more accurate, and some, such as the Insulet, Roche, and Animas systems, link with a meter that serves as a remote control for the pump.

One of the most significant "movements" in the pump industry is the integration of the insulin pump with a continuous glucose sensor. Currently, only one pump (Medtronic) displays sensor data on the pump screen, but other companies are in the process of linking with sensors as well. This eliminates the need to carry a separate device to display sensor data and integrates historical data into one convenient place.

More importantly, progress is being made in "closed loop" technology, whereby the pump makes insulin delivery decisions on its own based on input from a continuous glucose sensor. Medtronic's Veo pump, already available in many countries outside the United States, features an automatic pump delivery shut-off if the user fails to respond to a low glucose alert. This feature suspends basal insulin delivery for up to two hours, or until the glucose reaches a safe level. Research has shown that this feature is effective for circumventing severe hypoglycemia without resulting in severe high blood sugar or ketoacidosis.

Advanced features aside, the qualities/skills that are most important for those considering an insulin pump are:

- Motivation or interest in going on a pump, keeping in mind that nobody is 100 percent sure that it is right for them until they give it a try.
- adequate resources to afford the pump and ongoing supplies (via insurance or cash).
- the ability to count grams of carbohydrate in meals and snacks.
- monitoring blood glucose at least four times daily.
- record-keeping in paper or electronic form.
- ability to self-adjust insulin doses.
- an understanding of the basic principles of basal/bolus insulin therapy.

Successful pump use will also require adequate follow-up and fine-tuning. This should include careful adjustment of basal and bolus settings, troubleshooting guidelines, and education on how to utilize the pump's advanced features.

Selecting a pump is as much about personal preference as it is about technical specs. All pumps have a set of basic features that allow safe, precise delivery of basal and bolus insulin. Beyond that, a variety of features and characteristics make some pumps more appealing to certain people. Since you'll likely be using the same pump for many years, it pays to shop around for the pump with the features you desire.

✳ Trend

The type of pump should be chosen by the person who will be using it, not his or her physician.

The features that are important to consider when selecting a pump include:

- **Reservoir Volume** Does it hold enough insulin to last you at least three days (the typical cycle for infusion set changes)?
- **Readability** Is the screen bright and sharp enough for you to read the details easily?
- **Bolus Amounts** Are the bolus dose ranges (largest and smallest) suitable to your needs?
- **Calculation Features** Does the pump's bolus calculator allow you to enter your exact dosing formulas (insulin-to-carb ratios, target blood glucose, correction factors, duration of insulin action) without having to round off or compromise?

- **Alarms** Can you hear or feel the alarms when they go off?
- **Water Resistance** Do you require a pump that is fully waterproof?
- **Linkage** Do you want or need a pump that links electronically to a blood glucose meter or continuous glucose monitor?
- **Wearability** Is the size of the pump and clip/attachment configured well for you?
- **Coverage** Does your health insurance only cover certain pumps, or is the choice yours?

To learn more about pump therapy, contact one of the insulin pump manufacturers listed below or talk with your physician or diabetes educator. Find out if there are insulin pump user groups in your area. Group meetings offer an excellent forum for meeting other pumpers and finding out about their personal experiences since starting pump therapy.

Pump Manufacturers:
- Animas Corp. (Ping insulin pumps)
  877-937-7867; www.animascorp.com
- Asante Solutions (Pearl Insulin Pump)
  408-716-5600; www.asantesolutions.com
- Insulet Corp. (OmniPod)
  800-551-2475; www.myomnipod.com
- Medtronic Diabetes (Paradigm Revel insulin pumps)
  800-646-4633; www.medtronicdiabetes.net
- Roche/Disetronic (Accu-Chek Combo system)
  800-280-7801; www.accu-chekinsulinpumps.com

• Tandem Diabetes (t:slim insulin pump)
  877-801-6901; www.tandemdiabetes.com

"OTHER" MEDICATIONS

Many people feel that just because they take insulin, all the other diabetes medications just "aren't for them." Whether you have type 1 or type 2 diabetes, the "other" medications hold a great deal of potential for helping you improve your diabetes control and improve your quality of life.

Sadly, most primary-care physicians are not up-to-date, experienced, or comfortable with all of the latest medications that are available. You owe it to yourself to understand all you can about diabetes medications. The more you know, the better you can participate in your own care and ask the right kinds of questions. **Never hesitate to make a suggestion to your physician.** Just make sure it's based on sound information and presented in a collaborative way.

New Injectable Meds

Diabetes medications come in two forms: pills and injectables. By now, you're all too familiar with one of the injectables—insulin. Since its discovery back in the 1920s, insulin has been the only injectable treatment for diabetes, and the only treatment for type 1 diabetes, until recently.

Amylin

The first non-insulin injectable to hit the market was pramlintide (brand name Symlin), a replacement for the amylin hormone that is normally secreted by the pancreas along with insulin. People with type 1 diabetes secrete no amylin at all, and people with type 2 diabetes secrete far too little.

What's so important about amylin? Plenty. Whereas insulin regulates the removal of glucose from the bloodstream, amylin regulates its appearance. To be specific, amylin does the following:

- Slows the emptying of the stomach's contents into the small intestine, thus producing a more gradual blood sugar rise after meals.
- Blunts the secretion of glucagon by the pancreas (ironically, the pancreas of people with diabetes secretes extra glucagon just after meals), thus reducing post-meal blood sugar spikes and overall basal insulin needs.
- Enhances satiety and decreases appetite, thus lowering the amount of food that is raising the blood sugar.

Besides making blood sugar easier to manage, Symlin can also be a valuable weight-loss tool. Users of Symlin lose an average of more than 6 pounds. (2.5 kg) over the first 6 months of use, mainly by consuming smaller portions at meals and snacking less often. Given that many people with diabetes have difficulty controlling their appetite, Symlin has obvious lifestyle benefits. Symlin is intended for people on basal/bolus insulin programs. It will not eliminate the need for insulin, but it usually reduces the required doses.

✳ Trend

Symlin can be effective for countering post-meal blood sugar spikes and overeating in those on intensive insulin programs.

On the downside, Symlin's effects only last for about three hours, so it needs to be injected at just about every meal in order to work throughout the day. It is administered in the same manner as insulin: injected into the subcutaneous fat using a pen device. It cannot be mixed with insulin because it is slightly acidic, which causes it to sting a bit when injected.

The most common side effect associated with Symlin is nausea. Once a therapeutic dose is achieved, mild nausea (sometimes called "sour stomach") may occur 30 to 60 minutes after injection. This nausea tends to last for about 30 minutes and usually dissipates entirely after a few weeks as the body becomes re-acclimated to having the amylin hormone present again.

Treating hypoglycemia can also present a challenge when using Symlin. During its peak action time (30 to 60 minutes after injection), Symlin blocks the secretion of glucagon and slows digestion considerably. Attempts to treat hypoglycemia during this time may be unsuccessful. As a result, special efforts must be made to prevent hypoglycemia when taking Symlin. For those who take insulin at mealtimes, it may be necessary to reduce or delay the doses.

GLP-1

Whenever we eat food that contains carbohydrates (sugar or starch), some of the sugar comes in contact with the inner lining of the small intestine. When this happens, special chemical messengers are secreted by cells of the intestine. One of these chemical messengers, called glucagon-like peptide-1 or GLP-1 for short, helps the pancreas to release a rapid burst

The Bottom Line

Symlin is not for those looking to take a "casual" approach to diabetes management. It takes considerable effort to use Symlin successfully. But once the program is set up properly, the benefits can be significant. Symlin may be the most potent tool for controlling after-meal blood sugar levels, and is very effective at curbing hunger and preventing "grazing" and overeating. However, one must be willing to work through the nausea as well as the process of adjusting the doses of Symlin and mealtime insulin.

of insulin, decreases other hormones that raise blood sugar levels, slows digestion, and decreases appetite. GLP-1 does not promote low blood sugar or weight gain. Insulin secretion increases only when blood sugars are high and decreases as blood sugars approach normal.

Studies have shown that GLP-1 improves and preserves the health of the insulin-producing beta cells in the pancreas. Since progressive loss of these cells is an underlying cause of type 2 diabetes, GLP-1 has the potential to halt or reverse this process.

GLP-1 is available in three injectable forms: a twice daily (exenatide, brand name Byetta); a once daily (liraglutide, brand name Victoza); and a once weekly (exenatide extended release, brand name Bydureon). All are administered by way of a pen device. There are subtle differences in the way each works, so talk with your physician about the option that would best meet your needs.

GLP-1 can be used alone or in combination with oral diabetes medications or basal insulin. Many people also use it in combination with a basal/bolus insulin program, although this must be agreed upon by your physician. For those with type 1 diabetes, GLP-1 will not eliminate the need for insulin, but it will likely reduce it. For those with type 2 diabetes, it may reduce or eliminate the need for insulin or medication.

Varying degrees of nausea are common during the first few weeks of GLP-1 usage, but this usually subsides over time. Those with gastrointestinal problems or kidney disease are not usually good candidates for Symlin. The pens used to inject GLP-1 utilize very small disposable needles. The Bydureon injection requires a special mixing and syringe-filling process before the weekly injections can be administered.

> **✱ Trend**
>
> *GLP-1s offer multiple benefits to people with type 1 or type 2 diabetes.*

New Diabetes Pills

The newest of the oral diabetes medications are called **DPP-4 inhibitors.** We described above how GLP-1, produced by intestinal cells in response to a meal, is really good stuff for helping to control blood sugar levels. Unfortunately, GLP-1 only lasts for a few minutes because it is broken down by an enzyme called DPP-4. The job of a DPP-4 inhibitor is just that—to keep DPP-4 from breaking down GLP-1. This allows GLP-1 to circulate longer and work harder. And (perhaps) best of all, DPP-4 inhibitors do this without requiring an injection.

The Bottom Line

Despite having to be taken by injection and the short-term nausea experienced by many users, GLP-1 has the potential to offset many of the factors that contribute to elevated blood sugar. Its ability to facilitate weight loss is unmatched by any other diabetes medication. Individual responses to GLP-1 are highly varied—it works very well for some people, but seems to provide little benefit for others. You'll never know until you give it a try.

The currently available versions include sitagliptin (brand name Januvia), linagliptin (brand name Tradjenta), saxagliptin (brand name Onglyza) and vildagliptin (brand name Galvus). These can be taken in combination with other diabetes medications but must be used very carefully by those with poor kidney function. While DPP-4 inhibitors have been proven effective for improving blood sugar without causing hypoglycemia, they have not been shown to promote weight loss.

The Bottom Line

Given that they come in pill form, have minimal side effects, and can improve blood sugar levels significantly, DPP-4 inhibitors are becoming major players in diabetes treatment. They are the only oral diabetes medications that actually promote the growth and function of insulin-producing cells in the pancreas.

New Applications for Old Medications

Oral diabetes medications have been around for many decades. Researchers and clinicians have learned a great deal about their long-term effects and the potential some hold for treating other conditions. While the use of some diabetes pills is being curtailed, the use of others is expanding.

On the Rise: Metformin

Since being introduced in 1994, metformin (brand names Glucophage, Glucophage XR, Riomet liquid) has become the most widely prescribed medication for diabetes and one of the most widely used drugs in the world. Metformin does not increase insulin levels and does not cause hypoglycemia. Instead, it decreases the amount of

✱ Trend

Almost everyone with diabetes (including those with type 1 who are also insulin resistant) can benefit from metformin.

sugar produced by the liver and tends to suppress appetite. Secondary benefits may include improvements in cholesterol levels and insulin sensitivity. Metformin is often used in combination with other diabetes drugs or insulin, but it can also be effective when used alone. It should not be used by people with kidney impairment and should be used with caution by those with liver problems. Those who drink excessive amounts of alcohol should not use metformin. Potential side effects include upset stomach or a rare but serious condition called lactic acidosis (particularly when used by those with impaired liver function).

The Bottom Line

Because the liver is responsible for causing blood sugar to rise overnight, metformin can work quite well for those prone to elevated blood sugars upon waking. It can also reduce basal insulin needs for those taking insulin, which in turn can aid weight loss efforts. Side effects are minimal compared to other types of diabetes medication.

On the Rise: Combination Medications

One of the greatest obstacles to disease management is missed or neglected medication due to the complexity of one's program. By combining more than one medication into one pill, "combo meds" help to address this issue. With fewer pills to take and a simpler medication schedule, compliance almost always improves.

Several combination pills are currently available:
- Glucovance is a combination of glyburide (a sulfonylurea) and metformin.
- Avandamet is a combination of rosiglitazone (an insulin sensitizer) and metformin.
- ActoplusMet is a combination of pioglitazone (an insulin sensitizer) and metformin.
- Metaglip is a combination of glipizide (a sulfonylurea) and metformin.
- Avandaryl is a combination of rosiglitazone (an insulin sensitizer) and glimepiride (a sulfonylurea)

- Duetact is a combination of pioglitazone (an insulin sensitizer) and glimepiride (a sulfonylurea)
- Janumet is a combination of sitagliptin (a DPP-4 inhibitor) and metformin

The Bottom Line

Combination pills are purely a matter of convenience, and most include older-generation medications that are less effective than the new ones. But if you need to take a multitude of pills, there's nothing wrong with a little simplicity.

On the Decline: Pancreatic Stimulators (Sulfonylureas and Meglitides)

The very first medications used to treat type 2 diabetes targeted the pancreas directly by increasing the release of insulin. One class of these medications is called **sulfonylureas**. Older generations of these drugs include chlorpropamide (Diabinese), tolazamide, and tolbutamide. Newer sulfonylureas include glyburide (DiaBeta, Glynase, Micronase), glipizide (Glucotrol, Glucotrol XL), and glimepiride (Amaryl). These drugs work for 12 to 24 hours (or more, in the case of the older drugs) to lower blood sugar. Because sulfonylureas increase insulin production regardless of need, there is a risk of developing hypoglycemia (low blood sugar). Common side effects include weight gain, skin rash, and upset stomach. In addition, sulfonylureas are sulfa-containing drugs and should be avoided by people who have sulfa allergies.

A newer class of medications that stimulate pancreatic insulin production is called meglitinides. Drugs in this class include repaglinide (Prandin) and nateglinide (Starlix). Like sulfonylureas, meglitinides also work on the pancreas to promote insulin secretion. However, unlike sulfonylureas (which work gradually over an extended period of time), melgitinides are very short acting, with peak effects within one hour. For this reason, they are usually taken two or three times a day, just before meals, and are effective for controlling after-meal blood sugar levels. Meglitinides may cause hypoglycemia and weight gain, but these are less common than with sulfonylureas because of their shorter duration of action. Meglitinides may be safe to use with poor kidney function, but should not be used by people with liver disease.

* Trend

Use of sulfonylureas is on the decline because they wear out the pancreas prematurely, and better alternatives are now available.

On the Decline: Insulin Sensitizers (Thiazolidinediones)

Thiazolidinediones, also called TZDs, are medications that increase the sensitivity of the body's muscle and fat cells to insulin. TZDs include pioglitazone (Actos) and rosiglitazone (Avandia). Both pioglitazone and rosiglitazone act quickly and are usually taken once daily, but it may take six to twelve weeks for them to start having a significant effect on blood sugar levels. Both may be used in combination with other oral diabetes drugs as well as insulin. Both medications, but

The Bottom Line

Sulfonylureas and meglitinides are of no use to people with type 1 diabetes. They are usually effective for lowering blood sugar levels in those who are in the very early stages of type 2 diabetes, before the pancreas has lost the ability to secrete sufficient amounts of insulin. However, by increasing the workload on the pancreas, these drugs may actually accelerate its breakdown.

One must be very careful not to miss meals when using sulfonylureas due to the risk of hypoglycemia. For those with high blood sugar levels after meals, meglitinides offer more benefits and fewer risks. Because both types of medications tend to cause weight gain, extra emphasis must be placed on healthy lifestyle habits.

pioglitazone in particular, may offer an added benefit of raising HDL (good) cholesterol levels and lowering triglycerides.

There is a risk of developing liver problems with use of these drugs, so liver function tests are often taken during the first year of use. People with existing liver disease should not use these medications. Fluid retention can also occur (particularly with rosiglitazone) so people with poor heart function or a history of congestive heart failure are also not good candidates for TZDs. Sometimes, a diuretic (water pill) is needed to reduce fluid retention compounded by use of these drugs. Other potential side effects include anemia and an increased risk of bone fractures.

The Bottom Line

TZDs held a great deal of promise when they were first introduced because they tackle diabetes at the source: insulin resistance. Those who are extremely obese but otherwise healthy can certainly benefit from improving their insulin sensitivity. Recently, the possibility of heart complications associated with TZD use has discouraged many clinicians from prescribing them. And the fact remains: you can gain similar benefits to TZDs simply by exercising and eating right, but without the potential side effects.

On the Decline: Digestion Blockers (Alpha-Glucosidase Inhibitors)

Before being absorbed into the bloodstream, carbohydrates must be broken down into smaller sugar molecules, such as glucose, by enzymes in the small intestine. One of the enzymes involved in breaking down carbohydrates is called alpha-glucosidase. By inhibiting this enzyme, carbohydrates are not broken down as efficiently and glucose absorption is delayed. Alpha-glucosidase inhibitors include acarbose (Precose) and miglitol (Glyset). When used alone, these medications are not as effective as most other medications for diabetes. But when used with other medications, such as sulfonylureas, they tend to produce better blood sugar control than sulfonylureas used alone, particularly after meals. Acarbose and miglitol are usually taken with each meal.

Because of the way they work, significant gastrointestinal side effects tend to occur. Abdominal pain, diarrhea, and gas are seen in up to 75 percent of users. Most of the gastrointestinal symptoms subside over the course of a few weeks, although many people report persistent problems. Acarbose and miglitol should not be used by people with bowel/intestinal conditions, kidney disease, or liver disease. Complex carbohydrates should not be used to treat hypoglycemia when taking acarbose or miglitol since they will digest very slowly; only simple carbohydrates such as glucose tablets should be used.

The Bottom Line

Acarbose and miglitol may provide some help for those who experience blood sugar spikes after meals that are heavy in complex carbohydrates. And since they don't cause hypoglycemia and may diminish the between-meal appetite, they could be a boon to those trying to lose weight. However, the side effects are more than most people are willing to endure. Many people just don't make it past the "adjustment" phase of these drugs before calling it quits.

Chapter Four

Monitoring and More

Those in the know say that information is power. A healthy pancreas (technically, a healthy beta cell) collects and uses information constantly. A slight increase in glucose levels triggers the release of stored-up insulin and amylin. A slight decrease stops the release. It's this kind of automatic regulation that allows people without diabetes to focus their time and energy on things other than blood sugar control.

Central to the regulation of blood sugar is the collection and use of information ... namely blood glucose levels. Considerable improvements have been made in the way we measure blood sugar and collect/analyze the data. And even more amazing developments are just on the horizon. This chapter focuses on recent improvements in blood sugar measurement and data management technology.

POINT-IN-TIME BLOOD SUGAR MEASUREMENT

I can still remember my first blood glucose monitor, circa 1985. It was the size and weight of a brick and ran on a nine-volt battery. The test strips had a square application area (I still haven't figured out how to get a square drop of blood from my finger) that required a whopping 15-microliter sample. The testing procedure involved coding, blotting, wiping, and timing and took more than two minutes.

Even more fun was the lancing device—a medieval tool of torture that swung a thick 25-gauge lancet around in a half-circle toward my poor finger. Ouch!

Today's point-in-time blood glucose management tools have come a long, long way. We call them point-in-time to differentiate them from the various forms of continuous glucose monitoring systems that are now available. A point-in-time system is just what it sounds like—a glucose measurement that is provided at a specific moment in time, without consideration of the rate of change or trend.

Blood Glucose Meters

Let's look first at the current state and trends in blood glucose meters. Accuracy has always been an important criterion by which meters are evaluated, but today there is little difference in accuracy amongst the major systems. The differences lie in the convenience and usability features. While there is no single glucose meter that does everything for everyone, each one has its own unique features. It is to your advantage to find a meter that has

✳ Trend

With the frequency of blood glucose monitoring on the rise, it is more important than ever to find a meter with features that best meet your personal needs.

the combination of features that are most important to you.

People with type 1 diabetes are checking blood sugar more often than ever. Consumer research conducted by Children With Diabetes (a division of the Johnson & Johnson Company) has shown that the self-reported frequency of blood glucose checks has increased from four to more than seven times per day in just the past ten years.

Speed The time it takes for the meter to produce a reading is important because we all have things to do besides tending to our diabetes. And the more often you check, the more important it is to have a fast meter. In fact, if you check your blood sugar just four times daily, switching from a meter that takes 15 seconds to one that takes 5 seconds will save you more than four hours per year just waiting for readings to appear!

Currently, the fastest systems on the market are the WaveSense meters from AgaMatrix (4 seconds), FreeStyle and Precision meters from Abbott (5 seconds), Contour meters from Bayer (5 seconds), Nova Max meters from Nova Biomedical (5 seconds), OneTouch meters from LifeScan (5 seconds), and Accu-Chek meters from Roche (5 seconds).

Meter Size As long as your vision is good, smaller is usually better. It is important that meters be portable so that levels can be checked anytime, anywhere. However, also keep in mind that the size of the test strip vial and lancing device will affect how much you need to carry.

The iBGStar from Sanofi-Aventis is extremely small and can be used independently or while plugged in to an iPhone or iPod. Other compact meters include the FreeStyle Lite from Abbott, Contour USB from Bayer, Accu-Chek Nano from Roche, and UltraMini from LifeScan. The Precision Xtra from Abbott is an average size, but the test strips are individually foil-wrapped, so this makes the full system more compact.

Blood Volume Sample size matters as well. The less blood a meter requires, the easier (and less painful) it is to obtain the blood sample, and the less likely you are to waste a strip due to under-dosing. For those who prefer to obtain a blood sample at an "alternate site" (forearm, leg, etc.), it is best to use

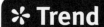

> ✳ **Trend**
>
> *Today, most meters use no more than ½ microliter of blood and take no longer than 5 seconds to provide a reading.*

a meter that requires 0.5 microliters (µl) of blood or less.

Systems with the smallest blood requirement include FreeStyle meters from Abbott (0.3 µl), Nova Max meters from Nova Biomedical (0.3 µl), Verio from LifeScan (0.4 µl), WaveSense meters from AgaMatrix (0.5 µl), and iBGStar from Sanofi-Aventis (0.5 µl).

Simplicity Most current meters require no coding (test strips are manufactured under uniform conditions) and do not require any button presses to do a basic blood glucose check—just insert the strip and apply the drop. Some meters have multiple test strip "packets" integrated into the meter so that strips don't have to be inserted into the meter every time you check. The Accu-Chek Compact Plus from Abbott and Ascensia Breeze2 from Bayer have this feature. The Accu-Chek Compact Plus also integrates the lancing device into the side of the meter, giving it a true all-in-one advantage.

Display Many meter manufacturers are moving toward interactive screens that are easier for the user to read. Color screens can be found on the Verio from LifeScan and Contour USB from Bayer. The Contour USB and Accu-Chek Compact Plus and Nano from Roche are also quite bright and offer excellent screen contrast. The InsuLinx from Abbott is the first to incorporate touch-screen technology for performing meter programming and reviewing data in the meter's memory.

Voice Capability For those with very limited (or no) vision, a talking meter allows for much greater independence. The "Voice" meter from Prodigy features audible messages and specially imprinted buttons. The "AutoCode" meter from Prodigy features audible messages and does not require coding for each new vial of strips.

Logging Capability The ability to record more than just glucose values can turn any meter into a full record-keeping system. Many meters allow the user to "tag" readings as pre- or post-meal, but some allow for the entry of more detailed information, such as food/carbs, exercise, and insulin/medication doses. These include InsuLinx from Abbott, OneTouch UltraSmart from LifeScan, and Accu-Chek Complete from Roche.

Data Analysis/Feedback It's one thing to perform blood glucose checks, but it's another thing entirely to gather the data, analyze it, and form conclusions that can be used to improve control. The use of download software will be discussed later in this chapter, but even that requires a computer or PDA and some technical expertise. While virtually all meters are downloadable to a computer, some

—including Contour USB from Bayer and InsuLinx from Abbott—have simplified the process by incorporating "plug and play" technology. The software for downloading the meter is built into the meter itself.

Another meter, the Verio from LifeScan, provides automated feedback based on recent glucose values. If a trend of above- or below-target readings is detected over a period of multiple days, a message is displayed.

Remote Transmission For those who use insulin pumps and utilize the pump's bolus "calculator" to determine insulin doses, it helps to have a meter that communicates directly with the pump. The OneTouch UltraLink from LifeScan, NovaMax Link from Nova Biomedical, and Contour Next Link from Bayer send radio transmissions to Medtronic Paradigm insulin pumps. The OneTouch Ping from LifeScan syncs with the Animas Ping insulin pump for purposes of calculating and programming boluses. The Accu-Chek Aviva Combo calculates bolus doses and uses Bluetooth technology to enter bolus doses into the Accu-Chek Combo pump. The Aviva Combo can also be used to program virtually all aspects of the Combo pump. The remote programmer for the OmniPod insulin pump system has a FreeStyle meter (from Abbott) built in. And the CoZmonitor from Abbott attaches to the back of the Deltec Cozmo insulin pump, transmitting the reading into its infrared ports.

Cost Savings Typically, as technology improves and becomes more widely used, the cost tends to come down. Unfortunately, this has not been the case with blood glucose meters. The meters themselves cost about the same as they did 20 years ago, and test strip costs have actually increased.

The good news is that most meter manufacturers provide medical offices with a large supply of samples to pass along to patients, and many offer co-pay assistance cards to help offset the ongoing cost of test strips. Ask your health-care provider for samples and co-pay cards if your health insurance does not cover the supplies you need.

Lancing

Getting a drop of blood may be the single most anxiety-provoking, inconvenient, and uncomfortable aspect of diabetes management. This is why literally billions of dollars have been invested in devices that can measure blood glucose levels without having to prick the skin. Unfortunately, none of these has come to fruition, and chances are they never will.

The good news is that we've come a long way since the "guillotine" device with the thick, painful lancets of yesteryear. Obtaining an adequate drop of blood with minimal discomfort is all about having the right tools and using the proper techniques. Lancets, like syringe needles, come in

> ✴ **Trend**
>
> *The days of painful finger-sticks are over. Use of very thin lancets, adjustable lancing devices, and alternate site testing should make blood sugar checks barely noticeable.*

varying gauges. The larger the gauge, the thinner (and less painful) they are. Look for lancets that are 33 gauge (or higher). Lancets as thin as 36 gauge are available for very young children from a company called, appropriately, "TiniBoy" (www.tiniboy.com).

And whatever you do, don't just poke your finger with the lancet by hand. Doing so virtually guarantees a painful fingerstick and buildup of scar tissue on your finger. Use a lancing device that has an adjustable depth setting. Start with the lowest/shallowest depth possible and see if you can conjure up a sufficient drop of blood … with a little bit of "milking." If that doesn't work, go to the next setting and so on until you obtain a sufficient drop. That's the setting you should go with and not a speck deeper. For alternate site testing, it is best to use a lancing pen that has a clear cap, so that you can see when a sufficient drop appears, and a thinner head than those used on the fingertips.

For those who prefer not having to change lancets often or deal with sharp objects, Roche has developed the Multiclix lancing device. The disposable head on the Multiclix contains six built-in lancets that rotate into position with each subsequent use. After activation, the lancets retract back into the head so that there is no risk of accidental needle sticks.

Lancing devices that minimize vibration and withdraw the lancet quickly after activation are also reported to improve user comfort. The Accu-Chek FastClix from Roche and OneTouch Delica from LifeScan incorporate these features.

CONTINUOUS GLUCOSE MONITORING

Point-in-time glucose readings are valuable. They allow us to calculate appropriate insulin doses, evaluate what we did previously, and fix elements of the diabetes management program that aren't working as well as they should. Like a photograph, they show what is currently going on, but they don't provide context.

Adding a continuous glucose monitor (CGM) is like taking those photographs and turning them into a movie, complete with "story notes." Now we can learn the full story. Today's CGMs display updated glucose information every five minutes. They also provide trend graphs, warning alerts, and downloadable reports.

Currently, CGM systems are available from two companies: Medtronic and Dexcom. Abbott also offers a CGM system called Navigator in some countries outside the United States. Medtronic offers a stand-alone system called Guardian, as well as a sensor/transmitter system that links with certain Medtronic insulin pumps. Dexcom's current system, the G4 Platinum, is a stand-alone system; no pump or other special equipment is required. However, most insulin pump companies have already announced their intention to incorporate a receiver and display for the Dexcom G4 in their next-generation pumps.

Some medical offices make use of something called "Professional" CGM systems, as opposed to the "Real-Time" systems that patients purchase for daily personal use. Professional systems are worn for a fixed period of time (typically three days) with the user unable to see the data while they wear it. Health-care providers download the professional system after removing it from the patient in order to look for patterns and trends that can be used to make therapy adjustments.

Regardless of the system, all CGMs include a flexible metallic filament inserted just below the skin to detect glucose in the interstitial fluid (fluid between fat cells). The information from the sensor is transmitted via radio signals to a handheld receiver that (except with professional systems) displays an estimate of the current glucose level. The user can set the receiver to provide alerts, by way of beeps or vibrations, when the glucose level is above or below target.

In some cases, the sensor information can be displayed right on an insulin pump. Data from the Medtronic sensor can be displayed on Medtronic insulin pumps (model x22 and higher), and data from the Dexcom sensor can display on the Animas Vibe pump (available only in certain countries outside the United States). All CGM systems require occasional calibration by way of fingerstick readings. Even though they are not as precise as blood glucose meters (the sensors are generally within approximately 15 percent of fingerstick values), they still offer considerable value to the user.

One of the key benefits of a CGM is the ability to detect approaching high or low glucose levels. CGMs provide a warning much earlier than most people can "feel" modest highs or lows on their own. This allows for early correction with food or insulin before extreme highs and lows develop. Essentially, this allows users to keep their glucose levels within their target range more often.

The on-screen trend graphs and directional arrows give users the ability to forecast where the glucose is headed so that appropriate decisions can be made regarding food, activity, and insulin/medication. For example, if you were about to exercise and knew that your glucose level was 150 mg/dl (8.3 mmol/l), you would probably act differently if you knew that it was dropping quickly as opposed to holding steady.

CGMs are downloadable for analyzing overall statistics and trends. The programs and equipment used will be discussed in more detail later in this chapter. The downloaded data can be used to:

- measure the magnitude of post-meal spikes
- test basal insulin doses
- evaluate post-meal and post-exercise patterns
- detect nighttime lows or rebounds
- measure the precise action curve for rapid-acting insulin
- determine the effectiveness of other medications
- evaluate responses to stress and illness

Research has shown that those who use their CGM consistently tend to have fewer and less severe episodes of hypoglycemia and improvements in their A1c, along with less variability in their glucose levels. Those who don't use them on a consistent basis may

✳ Trend

Many health professionals now recommend continuous glucose monitoring for the majority of their insulin-using patients.

benefit while wearing them but tend to see little in terms of long-term A1c improvements.

Health professional organizations recommend ongoing CGM usage for adults and children who use insulin, particularly those who:

- check their blood sugar regularly and are committed to intensive diabetes management
- have hypoglycemia unawareness or frequent hypoglycemia
- have considerable variability in their glucose levels

- require an HbA1c reduction without increased hypoglycemia
- are pregnant or planning pregnancy
- are athletes or engage in a high-risk profession

Why would anyone not use CGM all the time? Well, they do have a few drawbacks. Inserting the sensor can be a bit awkward and uncomfortable, and just having something stuck on the skin all the time bothers some people. There are periods of inaccuracy and occasional false alarms, and there is inherent "lag time" in any CGM system. Their readings lag about 10 minutes behind actual blood glucose values, so CGMs tend to read below actual blood glucose values when the blood sugar is rising, and above when blood sugar is falling. Transmitters and receivers require charging. Many people prefer not to carry around the receiver wherever they go. And finally, there are costs: even with insurance coverage, there are usually co-pays and deductibles that must be met.

The trend in CGM product development is quite positive. There is a growing movement toward linking the sensors and transmitters with devices such as insulin pumps, smart phones, and other common handheld devices. While Medtronic already links its sensor with its pumps, Dexcom is in the process of linking with various pumps and pump programmers. Dexcom's latest system features a much more robust transmitter with a wider broadcast range. This allows users (or

✳ Trend

There is a growing movement toward linking CGMs with insulin pumps and handheld devices such as cell phones and PDAs.

their caregivers) to be able to see data on the receiver even if the sensor is being worn in another room or across a sports field.

Medtronic recently introduced a bedside alarm clock-like device called mySentry. This device can be kept at the user's bedside or in the bedroom of a parent/caregiver. The mySentry device displays the data from the sensor on a large full-color screen and can trigger a powerful alarm in the event of system issues or glucose control problems.

Medtronic has also introduced a new sensor called Enlite in several countries outside the United States. The new sensor is shorter and much finer (thinner) than the current Sof-Sensor. It inserts at a right angle, perpendicular to the skin, and is considerably more comfortable to wear. The insertion process is also made less traumatic by using an automated insertion device that completely hides the introducer needle from the user.

To learn more about CGM and assistance with obtaining insurance coverage, there are several online resources that you can access:

The Juvenile Diabetes Research Foundation details the steps for obtaining case-by-case coverage for CGM at its website:
http://www.jdrf.org/index.cfm?page_id=107655

Sample letters for establishing medical need can be found at:
www.diabeteshealth.com/read/2009/02/27/6096/sample-request-for-cgm-insurance-coverage/

For additional resources for CGM insurance coverage,
visit the CGM Anti-Denial Campaign website:http://cgm-antidenial.ning.com

A comprehensive list of published articles supporting CGM use can be found at:
http://thecgmresourcecenter.com/cgm-library

RECORD-KEEPING AND DATA ANALYSIS PROGRAMS

What good is blood glucose data if it is not used to fine-tune one's program? Well, in order to use it in this way, the information must be collected and displayed in such a way that trends and patterns can be detected. Given the volume of data involved, and most people's general dislike for keeping written records, electronic record-keeping systems have grown in popularity.

Meter Downloading

Virtually all blood glucose meters are downloadable to a PC running in a Windows environment; many are also downloadable to a Mac. The meters themselves attach a time and date stamp to each glucose value so that graphs, charts, and statistics can be generated. Of course, it helps if the meter's clock and calendar are set properly, so check these before doing a download. If your meter allows you to "mark" readings as pre- or post-meal, these will also be listed, as will any additional information entered into your meter (such as insulin doses, carbohydrates, and exercise).

Meter downloading software is usually free of charge. It can often be downloaded from the meter company's web site or by obtaining the software on a CD. Download cables, which plug into your computer's USB port, are either free or modestly priced. Some meters connect directly to your computer; these usually have the download software built into the meter. Others use infrared or radio signals to communicate with your computer. Some of the newer meters connect directly to mobile devices that have applications for displaying the data.

Below is a summary of meter manufacturers and where to access the downloading materials:

Meter Maker	Web site	Phone Number
Abbott / FreeStyle	https://www.abbottdiabetescare.com/abbott-diabetes-care/products/patient/data-management.html	888-522-5226
AgaMatrix / WaveSense	http://www.wavesense.info/zero-click	866-906-4197
Bayer / Ascensia	http://www.winglucofactspro.com/	800-348-8100
LifeScan / OneTouch	http://www.lifescan.com/about-us	888-567-3003
Nipro Diagnostics	http://www.niprodiagnostics.com/our_products/ma_true_manager.aspx	800-803-6025
Nova Biomedical	http://www.novamaxlink.com/nova_max_link/	800-681-7390
Roche / Accu-Chek	https://www.accu-chek.com/us/data-management/360-software.html	800-858-8072

There are also programs that are independent of the meter and strip manufacturers. DiabetEASE (www.diabetease.com) is a free web-based program that lets users upload blood glucose readings and then generate graphs and charts for personal analysis. MyCareConnect (www.mycareconnect.com) is an online system that allows children to share their information with parents, teachers, nurses, and their health-care team while they are at school. Data can be entered on the web site or by text message, and all designated parties receive an instant update.

The Lowdown from the Downloads

Each software package offers its own unique set of reports. Most allow you to customize important factors such as your target blood glucose range and typical meal/snack times. Of the multitude of reports that can be generated, a few are particularly helpful.

The **Standard Day** or **Modal Day** report provides a scatter plot of blood glucose values arranged by time of day. It provides a quick visual summary of the blood glucose control at various mealtimes. Are there frequent highs or lows at certain times of day? Are the readings consistent or widely scattered?

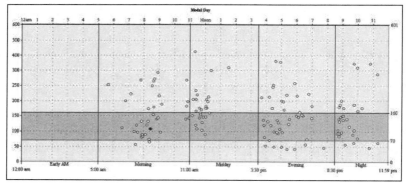

Example 1: Modal Day report from WinGlucofacts (Bayer/Ascensia)

Along with the Standard/Modal Day, a **Statistical Summary** can be quite useful. Statistical reports usually include glucose averages, standard deviations, and percentage of values above, below, and within the target range. They may also allow a breakdown of these values by time of day or day of the week. Statistical summaries provide a good measure of progress since the last time changes were made to your program.

Statistics Report
3/12/2008 - 4/11/2008

G Glucose Statistics (mg/dL)	Breakfast		Lunch		Dinner		Bed & Sleep		Total/Summary
	Pre	Post	Pre	Post	Pre	Post	Bed	Sleep	
#Readings	7	8	31	13	18	4	30	4	113
#Days w/Readings	7	8	26	13	18	4	24	4	31
Avg. # Readings/day	0.2	0.3	1.0	0.4	0.5	0.1	1.0	0.1	3.6
Highest	226	152	289	206	225	419	310	260	419
Lowest	71	98	65	116	112	141	79	117	66
Average	127	119	153	152	160	240	182	200	162
Standard Deviation	48.9	14.6	52.0	32.5	35.3	106.0	56.5	57.1	56.4
Above %	14	0	23	31	31	75	37	50	29
Within %	86	100	74	69	69	25	63	50	70
Below %	0	0	3	0	0	0	0	0	1

Example 2: Statistics Report from CoPilot Software (Abbott)

Glucose Trend Graphs provide a longitudinal plot of blood glucose values over an extended period of time, such as a month or several months. By highlighting periodic peaks and valleys, these graphs can help determine whether therapy adjustments are needed for factors such as weekends versus weekdays, pre- versus post-menstrual cycles, or variations in seasonal activity. Trend graphs are also useful for illustrating glycemic changes over prolonged periods of time.

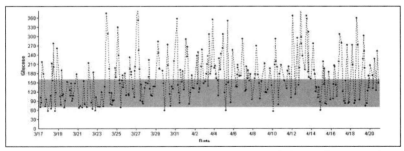

Example 3: Glucose Trend Graph from OneTouch DMS (LifeScan/OneTouch)

Logbook reports provide a listing, by time of day or mealtime, of glucose values so that you can learn about cause-and-effect relationships. Do your high readings come down to normal by the next time you check? Are highs preceded by lows? Are your readings different following physical activity? If your meter includes entries for items such as insulin doses, grams of carbohydrate, and physical activity, the logbook report can provide insight for fine-tuning things like insulin-to-carb ratios and exercise adjustments.

Legend		Breakfast			Lunch			Dinner			Bedtime	Night
		Before 5:00 AM-8:59 AM	Insulin	After 9:00 AM-9:59 AM	Before 10:00 AM-1:59 PM	Insulin	After 2:00 PM-5:59 PM	Before 6:00 PM-8:59 PM	Insulin	After 9:00 PM-9:59 PM	Insulin 10:00 PM-1:59 AM	2:00 AM-4:59 AM
F	12/16/11	366			235		164				288	
S	12/17/11			165	98 85		88				136	
S	12/18/11				145		72				260	
M	12/19/11	140 136			95		84				267	
T	12/20/11	198			100		216			84	411	
W	12/21/11	179 396			220						190	
T	12/22/11	119		81	270		148				399	
F	12/23/11			351	104						292 188	
S	12/24/11				136		66				109	131
S	12/25/11				125		120	177			309	
M	12/26/11				273					92	153	
T	12/27/11			253	143					211	98 104 226	

Example 4: Logbook report from Nova Diabetes Software

Pump Downloading

Most modern insulin pumps contain extensive information that can be used for pinpointing problem areas and revealing sources of problematic blood sugars. Historical information in pumps includes insulin delivery (both basal and bolus), daily insulin totals, blood glucose entries, carb entries, alarms/alerts, and priming of tubing and infusion sets.

Medtronic insulin pumps download wirelessly to a web-based program called CareLink (carelink.minimed.com). The downloading process requires a radio transmitter/receiver, either a CareLink USB device or a Contour Next Link meter, that plugs directly into the USB port of virtually any computer. One of these devices is included with most pumps when they ship out; they can also be purchased directly from Medtronic. In addition to reading Medtronic pump data, CareLink also reads data from a number of blood glucose meters as well as CGM data from Medtronic pumps and Guardian systems.

CareLink comes in two forms: Personal and Professional. The Professional version is primarily for health-care practices. CareLink Personal generates a number of useful reports, including a Logbook Diary (which provides details in super-imposed chronological order), Modal Day Periods (similar to a blood glucose modal day chart with statistics), Trend Summaries (showing average insulin, blood glucose and carb information over a period of time), and Device

✳ Trend

Increasingly, software programs for diabetes devices are moving toward web-based platforms. This allows users to download at home and share their data with health-care providers.

Settings (a complete report of pump settings). Users have the option of generating single reports or "batch" reports all at one time. And because the program is web-based, users can download at their home or office and then share their login ID with health-care providers, enabling them to view the data.

The Animas pump downloads to a web-based program called Diasend (diasend.com). Like CareLink, Diasend can integrate data from multiple devices (blood glucose meters, Dexcom CGM, Animas pump data) and generates many different types of reports, including Glucose Standard Day (for a blood sugar modal day chart), Insulin Pump Settings (for a complete listing of settings in the pump), Comparison Table (for comprehensive logsheets), and Compilation (for statistical summaries). Downloading requires an infrared interface cable that can be obtained from Animas.

The OmniPod programmer (PDM) and Deltec Cozmo insulin pumps download to the Copilot software program from Abbott https://www.abbottdiabetescare.com/abbott-diabetes-care/products/patient/data-management.html. However, in order to read data from the pumps, "extension" software must be added to the Copilot program. The extension software can be obtained from the pump manufacturer or on the pump company's web site. Downloading the OmniPod PDM requires a cable that plugs into the port on the top of the device; downloading the Cozmo requires an infrared device. Once downloaded, Copilot generates a multitude of customizable reports similar to those described above. Copilot also allows users to "share" their data with healthcare providers by synchronizing with Abbott's online server.

The Accu-Chek Combo system downloads wirelessly (using an infrared reader) to Accu-Chek 360 software to create a series of comprehensive reports.

CGM Downloading

Continuous glucose monitoring systems have limited capability to produce useful historical reports on their own display screens. Downloading is necessary for detecting patterns, trends, and statistics.

The Medtronic CGM systems, as mentioned above, download wirelessly to the web-based CareLink program via a CareLink USB radio receiver or via the Contour Next Link meter from Bayer. CareLink generates a series of reports incorporating the CGM data, including Daily Summaries (which include glucose data, insulin delivery, and carb entries for individual days), Sensor Daily Overlays (which superimpose up to seven days of sensor data for detection of repeated patterns), and Sensor Overlay By Meal (which, when used in conjunction with a Medtronic pump, shows after-meal glucose responses).

The Dexcom CGM downloads to the web-based Diasend program (described above for Animas pump downloading), as well as the company's own DM3 software. The latest Dexcom G4 Platinum downloads to Dexcom Studio software, available on the Dexcom web site. A cable plugs into the Dexcom receiver to transmit data to the computer. The software generates a variety of reports, including Glucose Trends (individual day reports that can include "events" that were entered into the receiver), Hourly Trends (average hourly statistics over a set period of time), Modal Day (superimposing multiple days' trend graphs for pattern detection), and a Success Report (statistical summaries comparing one time frame to the next). The data file from each download can be sent to health-care providers by e-mail. Providers can then import the data on a PC to perform an analysis.

Record Keeping "Apps"

For many years, we have known that record keeping improves individual performance and clinical outcomes. The trouble is, in today's "paperless" world, many people resist writing anything down! Luckily, there are other options: electronic diaries. The use of PDAs (personal digital assistants) was validated in a recent research study that showed that people who used PDAs to itemize their food intake were more likely to meet their dietary goals than those who used old-school handwritten diaries.

Use of diabetes applications (apps) for PDAs does more than just provide an organized set of records for analysis by you and your health-care team. It also makes everyone more accountable and responsible for their day-to-day actions. Most diabetes-related apps are made for the iPhone/iPad/iPod Touch devices, but some work with other devices as well. Here are a few examples:

The **iBG Star** Diabetes Management application from Sanofi Diabetes (www.ibgstar.us) seamlessly integrates with the iBGStar glucose monitor. Whenever you take a reading with your iBGStar while it is attached to your iPhone, the system automatically syncs your data with the iBGStar Diabetes Manager app. This app offers blood sugar tracking with tags (such as mealtimes and exercise), dynamic graphing, and sharing options.

The mobile phone application **dbees.com** (www.dbees.com) is a fully flexible and adaptable service for people with diabetes. In fact, the system itself selects the applicable activities and types of tests for each user's unique needs. It supports various forms of diabetes (type 1, type 2, gestational) and modes of treatment. Multiple languages are offered. It features customizable alarms and reminders. All data entered into your mobile phone are transferred to your online account where it can be accessed by you and your health-care team.

Diabetes 360 (diabetes360.deepbluewebtech.com) is designed for people of all ages with diabetes. This app includes an insulin dose calculator (based on the glucose level and total carbohydrate) as well as data logging and analysis. The carbohydrate database from the U.S. Department of Agriculture is on the iOS device (iPhone, iPod, iPad) so it can be accessed quickly whether there is network service available or not. Diabetes 360 can also handle simple sliding scales to calculate insulin dosing. There is a simple reminder system for pump site changes, meal/snack times, ketone checks, and long-acting insulin dosing. Log entries can be graphed and exported via e-mail to your health-care provider or imported as CSV files into a spreadsheet.

✳ Trend

Electronic record-keeping apps for mobile devices are becoming more widespread for tracking diabetes management activities.

Diabetes Pilot (www.diabetespilot.com) is a tool for managing diabetes on a variety of devices; versions are available for Mac, Desktop for Windows, iPhone/iPod Touch, Palm Handhelds, and Windows Mobile. It can be used alone or in combination with Diabetes Pilot Desktop software that works on Windows PCs and is sold separately. Information that you record on your mobile device can be transferred to Diabetes Pilot Desktop where reporting and printing features allow you to analyze your data, print it, back it up, and save it in various formats for e-mailing, faxing, and use in other programs. Diabetes Pilot includes an integrated food database and an insulin dose calculator for correcting high glucose readings and covering the carbohydrates, protein, and fiber in a meal based on parameters that you enter.

WaveSense Diabetes Manager (www.wavesense.info/iphone) is a free iPhone app from AgaMatrix. It lets you track blood sugars, insulin, and carbs. Data can be viewed in logbook or graphical format.

Glucose Buddy from SkyHealth (www.glucosebuddy.com) is a free iPhone app that allows for entry of blood sugars, insulin doses, carbs, and physical activities. Data are synced with a user account on the Glucose Buddy web site.

iRecordit from Communiteq Systems (www.irecordit.net) works on Blackberry mobile devices. It allows entry of a variety of lab results as well as blood sugars, meals, insulin doses, and physical activities. Reports can be viewed in a variety of formats and are easily shared by e-mail.

HOME LAB TESTING

It used to be that labwork could only be done ... well ... at a lab. Today, simple labwork involving small blood samples can be performed by everyday people using devices designed for home use.

Home A1c Kits

Currently, two companies offer A1c test kits for home use. Bayer's A1cNow SELFCHECK kit (www.a1cnow.com) is like a one-time-use blood glucose meter. Use it and then throw it away. A1c results are obtained in 5 minutes from a fingerstick blood sample. The procedure must be followed exactly according to the instructions in order to obtain results that are comparable to lab values.

The Appraise A1c Home Test from Heritage Labs is a collection kit that is mailed to the lab for analysis. Results are usually processed within three days of receipt of the sample. The test kit includes sample collection materials and a postage paid return envelope. For information, go to www.appraisetests.com or call 888-764-2384.

Ketone Testing

Measuring ketones in a urine sample is much like measuring glucose—delayed, imprecise, and inconvenient. Blood ketone measurement allows for rapid detection and accurate measurement of ketones so that corrective action can be taken.

Ketone testing is recommended at the first signs of (and during) illness, with unexplained hyperglycemia, during pregnancy, and prior to exercise when elevated glucose levels are present.

Abbott's Precision Xtra meter and Nova Biomedical's Nova Max Plus meter can measure ketones in a small blood sample in just a few seconds. Special ketone test strips must be used for performing these tests. Ketone measurements above 0.6 mmol/l are considered excessive; levels above 1.5 mmol/l are considered very dangerous.

Microalbumin

Not all trends in diabetes are for the better. Home microalbumin kits used to be available. These kits allowed individuals to perform basic screenings for early signs of kidney disease (nephropathy) by sending a urine sample to a lab for analysis. Unfortunately, these kits are no longer offered. Urine dipsticks such as the Micro Albumin 2-1 Combo Strip use color change to indicate the approximate amount of waste (creatinine) and protein (microalbumin) being excreted by the kidneys. High levels of microalbumin relative to creatinine have been identified as an early indicator of kidney problems. Early treatment is instrumental in slowing or stopping the progression toward kidney failure.

As we will discuss in the next chapter, aggressive screenings and early detection of diabetic complications are crucial to preventing serious disease and disability. With any luck, future editions of this book will include many more consumer products to assist us with these efforts.

Chapter
Five

Advances in Fighting Complications

Many of the decisions we make on a daily basis are made to simply put the odds in our favor. We get up and go to work to increase the chances that we won't get fired. We take the route to work that offers the best chances of getting there on time. And at lunchtime, we choose our foods to feel satisfied and (hopefully) keep us healthy long-term.

When we manage our diabetes, we are doing the same thing: playing the odds. As discussed back in chapter 1, keeping blood sugars near normal today helps us in countless ways to feel better and perform at our best. Over the long term, managing blood sugar gives us the best chances for preventing the serious health problems that plague so many people with diabetes—vision loss, kidney failure, nerve problems, and heart disease, just to name a few. We call these health problems "complications" because they stem from the diabetes.

Remember, playing the odds guarantees nothing. Just ask anyone who lost a lot of money investing in or betting on a "sure thing." While managing blood sugars effectively will certainly reduce your risk of developing complications, there is still the possibility that they can occur. The key is to catch them early and treat them aggressively so they don't have a major negative impact on your life. For example, there is a big difference between treating a damaged blood vessel in the back of your eye and losing your vision entirely.

This chapter is all about the latest developments in the prevention, detection, and treatment of diabetes complications. These developments benefit everyone with diabetes—whether your blood sugar control is way out of range or nearly perfect. They are just another way to increase your odds of living a long, healthy, happy life.

POSTPRANDIAL POWER

Before we discuss any specific complications, it is worth noting that, over the past several years, greater emphasis is being placed on blood sugar stability. It is normal for the blood sugar to rise a little bit after eating, but huge upswings followed by rapid downswings are a problem. It is difficult to maintain a tight A1c without paying attention to after-meal blood sugar levels. The long-term effects of after-meal highs (also called "postprandial" spikes) have been studied extensively. Significant post-meal rises have been shown to produce kidney disease at an earlier age and accelerate the progression of existing eye problems (retinopathy). And post-meal hyperglycemia is an independent risk factor for cardiovascular problems.

But the problems are not limited to long-term complications. Any time blood sugars rise particularly high, even temporarily, our quality of life suffers. Energy decreases, brain function falters, physical/athletic abilities become diminished, and moods become altered.

The reason blood sugar spikes so high after eating for many people with diabetes is a simple matter of timing. In most cases, food raises blood sugar much faster than rapid-acting insulin can lower it. For those who take rapid-acting insulin at meals, the result is a blood sugar spike 1 to 2 hours after eating.

Post-meal spikes can be measured in a variety of ways. Checking blood sugar about an hour after finishing a meal should provide a good indication of how much of a spike is taking place. Continuous glucose monitors provide trend graphs that make it easy to see exactly what is happening after meals. There is also a laboratory blood test called "GlycoMark" that measures the degree to which blood sugars are spiking over the past couple of weeks.

Different organizations have established different targets for after-meal blood sugar levels. However, it is best to develop an individualized set of goals with the guidance of your health-care team. In general, the following should serve as a good starting point:

Group/Age	Post-Meal Goal
Adults taking mealtime insulin	<180 mg/dl (10 mmol/l)
Adolescents (12-18)	<200 mg/dl (11)
School age children (6-11)	<225 mg/dl (12.5)
Preschool/Toddlers (≤5)	<250 mg/dl (14)
Women during pregnancy	<140 mg/dl (8)
Type 2s taking basal insulin only	<160 mg/dl (9)

To reduce post-meal spikes, a number of strategies can be used:

- Using rapid-acting insulin to cover meals and snacks, rather than regular insulin or NPH
- Taking mealtime insulin 15 to 30 minutes before eating
- Choosing foods that raise the blood sugar slowly; i.e., foods with low glycemic index values
- Adding vinegar to foods, since acidity slows the rate of digestion
- When having a mixed meal, consume the vegetables before the starchy portion of the meal
- Splitting meals into two or more parts, while still taking the full insulin dose before starting to eat the first portion
- Engaging in physical activity soon after eating
- If you use an insulin pump, replacing up to three hours of basal insulin with a bolus given at mealtime
- Utilizing an injectable incretin, such as Symlin, Byetta, Victoza, or Bydureon, to slow digestion and blunt the after-meal production of glucagon
- Preventing hypoglycemia before meals, since this accelerates the blood sugar rise from food
- If you have type 2 diabetes, using a meglitinide rather than a sulfonylurea due to its more rapid action, or using an alpha-glucosidase inhibitor to slow the absorption of sugars into the bloodstream

Now let's take a look at trends specific to the prevention, diagnosis, and treatment of the various complications of diabetes.

DIABETIC EYE DISEASE (RETINOPATHY)

The retina is the light-sensitive tissue in the back of the eye. It is common for blood vessels of the retina to become damaged over time when blood sugar levels are elevated. This is called diabetic retinopathy. Damaged blood vessels may leak blood into the clear fluid in the center of the eye, block light from reaching the light-sensitive tissue at the back of the eye, or keep adequate nutrients from reaching parts of the eye that are critical for normal vision. Elevated blood pressure also contributes to blood vessel damage.

Tight blood sugar and blood pressure control are priorities in the prevention of diabetic retinopathy. However, even with tight control, nothing is guaranteed. In the early stages of diabetic retinopathy, you may not notice any symptoms or changes to your vision. But over time, diabetic retinopathy tends to progress and cause vision loss, especially if it is not treated.

Early detection of diabetic retinopathy can, and does, lead to timely treatment and thus prevents vision loss. You should have the internal structures of your eyes checked regularly by an ophthalmologist or optometrist. It is necessary to dilate the pupils in order to examine the full retina. If the eyes are not dilated, the examiner will only be able to see the central portion of the retina (like the bulls eye on a target), but nothing else.

✳ Trend

Regular screenings and early detection of eye and kidney problems can prevent blindness and kidney failure in the majority of cases.

Every adult with diabetes should have a dilated eye exam immediately upon diagnosis of their diabetes, as eye problems may already exist. After the initial examination, screenings should be done every year, or more often if the eye doctor feels it is necessary.

Although diabetic retinopathy is rare in children prior to puberty, regular examinations are still recommended for pre-pubescent children, and annual examinations should be performed yearly after puberty. For women with type 1 diabetes who become pregnant, an immediate eye screening is essential. The hormonal and blood pressure changes that take place during pregnancy can speed up the progression of even very mild cases of retinopathy.

Treatment of retinopathy has become highly advanced in recent years. Laser treatment is one of the most effective tools used by ophthalmologists to prevent vision loss. A laser beam of light focused on weak or damaged blood vessels "seals" them so that they won't leak or hemorrhage. The focused laser procedure takes just a few minutes, and there is usually little or no discomfort. Laser treatment works best when retinopathy is caught early.

Another option used for treating diseases of the macula (the part of the retina responsible for central vision) is the use of injectable medications. Ranibizumab (brand name Lucentis) is used specifically for the treatment of macular degeneration and macular edema. Injected monthly, it inhibits the activity of growth factors that cause uncontrolled blood vessel growth and leakage in the eye. Clinical studies have shown significant vision improvements in the majority of patients who receive Lucentis injections.

DIABETIC KIDNEY DISEASE (NEPHROPATHY)

Nearly one out of three people with diabetes will eventually experience some form of kidney damage. When this occurs, the kidneys lose their ability to properly filter toxins out of the blood stream. This can easily be detected by measuring the level of creatinine and BUN in the blood. Unfortunately, by the time these substances are elevated, kidney disease has already reached a severe level and may progress to end-stage renal failure.

> **✳ Trend**
>
> *Blood pressure control is now emphasized almost as much as blood sugar control for the prevention of most complications of diabetes.*

In people with diabetes, long before toxins become elevated, the filtering units of the kidneys become "leaky" to protein. Special urine tests can be performed to detect early leakage of small amounts of protein, called "microalbuminuria." If you are found to have persistent microalbuminuria, you are at significant risk for developing severe kidney disease and need to be more attentive than ever to your overall health care.

In nearly all cases, kidney damage that is caught early can be slowed or halted. The most important factor is blood pressure control. People who have diabetes and microalbuminuria should attempt to keep their blood pressure below 130/80. Certain classes of blood pressure medications such as ACE inhibitors or angiotensin receptor blockers are most beneficial in protecting the kidneys and reversing or stabilizing microalbuminuria. Tight control of your blood pressure and cholesterol will also be beneficial in preserving your kidney function.

DIABETIC NERVE DISEASE (NEUROPATHY)

More than 50 percent of people with diabetes will develop some form of neuropathy. Peripheral sensory neuropathy causes tingling, numbness, pain, or hypersensitivity. Peripheral neuropathy often starts in the feet and moves its way up the legs. Motor neuropathies can cause muscle weakness, muscle wasting, and poorly coordinated movements. Autonomic neuropathies can lead to impaired digestion, bladder emptying problems, and sexual dysfunction. They can also cause heart rate/blood pressure abnormalities when sitting up or standing, as well as unusual sweating and difficulty with night vision.

Being diagnosed with neuropathy opens the door for potential treatments and strategies for preventing more severe problems. In some cases, the neuropathy may be related to a vitamin B12 deficiency, uncontrolled thyroid disease, rheumatologic problem, or other manageable conditions. Otherwise, treatment for neuropathy focuses on tight blood sugar control and management of symptoms. Painful diabetic neuropathies can now be treated with a variety of medications, including Lyrica (pregabalin), Neurontin (gabapentin), Effexor (vanlafaxine), Cymbalta (duloxetine), and amytriptiline. Alpha-lipoic acid, an over-the-counter antioxidant, has shown promise in a few studies, but not all. For some, neuropathic pain can be relieved by applying a lidocaine patch to the skin or using creams that contain a heat-releasing substance called capsaicin.

A number of non-medication alternative therapies may be helpful in select cases. These include use of foot tents, electrical nerve stimulation, acupuncture, biofeedback, and spinal cord stimulators. For those who smoke, quitting allows greater blood flow to nerve cells and may help reduce painful symptoms.

Perhaps the most publicized result of diabetic nerve disease is erectile dysfunction (ED). Erectile problems in men with diabetes are usually a result of both reduced blood flow and problems with the nerves that signal the opening of blood vessels in the penis. Given that ED affects tens of millions of men in the United States alone, treatment options have become a priority for the pharmaceutical industry. The introduction of sildenafil (Viagra) more than ten years ago was followed by vardenafil (Levitra) and tadalafil (Cialis). All three increase blood flow to the penis and permit relatively normal sexual intercourse for many users.

HEART DISEASE AND STROKE (MACROVASCULAR DISEASE)

Having diabetes raises the risk for heart attack and stroke, and the risk goes up right along with blood sugar, blood pressure, and cholesterol levels. Today, the emphasis is on not one, not two, but all three: The A, B, Cs so to speak. A for A1c (the lower the better, but certainly below 7 percent), the B for blood pressure (below 130/80), and the C for cholesterol (total below 180 and LDL below 100). In fact, these days it is common for physicians to prescribe blood pressure medications (usually ACE inhibitors) and cholesterol medications (usually statins) for people with diabetes whose levels are normal or slightly above normal, simply to offer extra protection against heart disease.

Because heart disease does not always cause chest pain (angina) in people who have a compromised nervous system, regular screenings for heart disease are in order for everyone with diabetes. Exercise stress tests performed every couple of years are a safe and excellent way to detect heart abnormalities that are still in a treatable phase—before they lead to a major heart attack or sudden death.

CIRCULATORY COMPLICATIONS (PERIPHERAL ARTERIAL DISEASE)

One in three people with diabetes over the age of 50 has some form of peripheral arterial disease (PAD), particularly affecting circulation in the legs. This can lead to slowly healing sores and painful cramping with exercise. Limited blood flow combined with a loss of nerve sensation in the extremities spells double trouble for the feet. Luckily, there are effective ways to prevent and treat PAD.

PAD screening should take place at least once every five years. This can be performed by your physician by comparing blood pressure in the ankle to blood pressure in the arm. Those diagnosed with PAD can increase their endurance and quality of life by engaging in a supervised walking program. Medications that reduce cholesterol and blood pressure and prevent blood clots can be effective for preventing as well as treating PAD. And more than ever, surgical procedures such as angioplasty (inflating constricted arteries with a tiny balloon) and bypass (creating alternate paths for blood to flow around blocked arteries) are providing relief for those with PAD.

GUM DISEASE (PERIODONTITIS)

A number of oral disorders are linked to diabetes, particularly periodontal (gum) disease. Interestingly, the relationship between diabetes and periodontal disease works both ways: Elevated blood sugar contributes to gum disease, and gum disease is associated with both high blood sugar and worsening of complications such as kidney and heart disease. One study showed that people who do not brush their teeth twice daily were 70 percent more likely to have a heart attack or other form of cardiovascular disease. Many people with poorly controlled diabetes also have reduced saliva production, which is associated with an increase in gum disease, tooth decay (cavities), and mouth infections.

Harmful plaque buildup above and below the gumline is a major underlying cause of gum disease. Frequent brushing, daily flossing, and regular cleaning by a dentist or dental hygienist have traditionally been keys to keeping teeth and gums healthy. In recent years, plaque removal has also been facilitated through the use of anti-plaque mouthwash and dental floss picks. Products that increase saliva production have also grown in popularity. Sucking on candies or chewing gum that contain xylitol has been shown to lower the risk of cavities. Lozenges containing essential oils (thymol, eucalyptol, and menthol) can be used by people with dry mouth to improve salivary flow. Recaldent (found in some chewing gums) has been shown to reduce acidity in the mouth and strengthen tooth enamel. In fact, use of sugarless gum of just about any type after meals is now endorsed by the American Dental Association as a means of reducing plaque and preventing cavities.

LIMITED JOINT MOBILITY

One of the less-recognized complications of diabetes involves tight or "frozen" joints—particularly in the shoulders and hands. Glucose, which sticks to almost everything it comes in contact with, also sticks to collagen—a protein found in abundance in cartilage and tendons. Glycosylation of collagen leads to stiffening and limited joint mobility. When this occurs in the hands, it is often called trigger finger. When it occurs in the shoulder, it is called adhesive capsulitis. Those who have been insulin dependent for many years seem to be particularly vulnerable.

Although most medicines (other than steroid injections) have come up short in preventing and treating joint mobility problems, some alternative therapies have proven to be quite effective. Physical therapy, performed early in the onset of symptoms, can help maintain joint strength and flexibility. And in a recent study, individuals with type 1 diabetes and frozen shoulder experienced significant improvement in shoulder comfort, function, and range of motion by participating in yoga sessions for 12 weeks.

Chapter
Six

The Latest
Resources

Taking care of diabetes is a demanding 24/7/365 job (366 during a leap year). Learning the latest strategies for self-management and keeping in stride with technology takes more than just seeing your doctor every couple of months. Even reading this book won't do it all. Web-based resources and other networking and educational opportunities make it possible for people with diabetes (PWDs) to live safely, successfully, and happily.

Getting the support one needs is a critical element of good diabetes care and positive outcomes. Research presented at the American Diabetes Association's Scientific Sessions in 2012 showed that increased social networking was associated with significantly lower HbA1c levels in teens and young adults with type 1 diabetes.

✳ Trend

More and more, people with diabetes are networking with their peers to share, learn, and commiserate about living successfully with diabetes.

In recent years, the Diabetes Online Community (DOC) has grown and flourished. There are literally hundreds of diabetes-focused web sites and blogs, each with a slightly different slant. PWDs and their caregivers are connecting around the world in various social media venues—providing opportunities to laugh, share, inform, motivate, sympathize, and, on occasion, simply amaze.

There are specialized blogs and web sites for those with particular areas of interest. For example:

Diabetes Advocates A collection of individuals and organizations that offer expertise, resources, and support to those touched by diabetes.
Web site: diabetesadvocates.org
Twitter: @D_Advocates

Diabetes Social Media Advocacy This community empowers, connects, supports, and educates PWDs. Check for twitter chats and DSMA live (talk radio).
Web site: http://diabetessocmed.com/
Twitter: @diabetessocmed, #dsma (hashtag)

Online Diabetes Communities Web sites where PWDs and loved ones are connecting. Popular sites include:

1happydiabetic.com/
Just the right formula for a positive attitude

bd.com/us/diabetes/page.aspx?cat=7001
BD (Becton-Dickinson)'s Diabetes Learning Center

childrenwithdiabetes.com
Unlimited resources for kids and parents

closeconcerns.com
A consultancy devoted to the business of diabetes

Collegediabetesnetwork.org
Networks of students with diabetes at colleges and universities

deo.ucsf.edu
University of California Online Diabetes Teaching Center

diabetesdaily.com
Diabetes news, tools, community, and blogs

diabetesincontrol.com
Free weekly news and information for diabetes health professionals

diabetesnet.com
Diabetes information, research findings, and discounted diabetes products

diabetessisters.org
Focused on women and women's issues

diabeticmommy.com
For expectant and recent moms

diabetesmine.com
A "Gold Mine" of straight talk and encouragement for people living with diabetes

diabeticinvestor.com
David Kliff's business/investor report on the diabetes industry (pay site)

diatribe.us/home.php
Research and product news for the "well-informed" person with diabetes

friendswithdiabetes.org
Incorporating diabetes into a Jewish lifestyle

hypoactive.org
Promoting an active lifestyle for PWDs in Australia

insulin-pumpers.org
For pump users and those interested in pump therapy

insulindependence.org
Inspiring fitness goals, adaptive strategies for sport, and recreational programs

juvenation.org
A network hub of type 1 diabetes communities, created by JDRF

mendosa.com/diabetes.htm
David Mendosa's web site (various resources and information)

myglu.org
For type 1s, sponsored by the Helmsley Trust

parentingdiabetickids.com
For parents of kids with diabetes

phrendo.com
Make personal connections with diabetic athletes

sixuntilme.com
Great sense of humor with Kerri Sparling

studentswithdiabetes.com
Organized by Nicole Johnson (Miss America 1999); provides a community for college students with diabetes

thebetesnow.com
Creative use of media in exploring the world of diabetes

thediabetesoc.com
Featured bloggers of the week

thediabetesresource.com
Your ultimate guide to everything diabetes related

triabetes.org

Athletes take on triathlons while mentoring "triabuddies"

tudiabetes.org

A Community of people touched by diabetes, run by the Diabetes Hands Foundation

www.type1university.com

The online school of higher learning for insulin users

Diabetes Blogs. There are almost as many diabetes blogs as there are PWDs. Popular ones include diabetesmine.com, diabetesaliciousness.blogspot.com, d-mom.com, huffington-post.com, sixuntilme.com, scottsdiabetes.com, textingmy-pancreas.com and many more:

25unitstogo.wordpress.com/

Harry's sarcastic outlook on life with diabetes

act1diabetes.org/

Blogs from various adults coping with type 1 diabetes

badpancreas.wordpress.com/

"Typical Type 1" Jacquie expresses herself in the most creative ways

christophermassa.blogspot.com/
A blog about photography and pushing one's self
through sport

www.d-mom.com/
The ups and downs of life with a diabetic child

diabetesaliciousness.blogspot.com/
Kelly Kunik tackles diabetes through humor, diabetes
ownership, and advocacy

diabetesdaily.com
A composite of many diabetes blogs

diabetesdaily.com/farrell/
Bernard Farrell's diabetes technology blog

diabetesstopshere.com
Blog of the American Diabetes Association

diabetesstories.com/stories_blog/
Author Riva Greenberg's inspiring and informative posts

diabetestalkfest.com
Gina Capone: Your Diabetes BFF

dorkabetic.blogspot.com
Hannah's dorky life with diabetes at

healthcentral.com/diabeteens/
Teen blog hosted by healthcentral

lemonlemonade.wordpress.com/
The journey of Allison Blass and her life with type 1 diabetes

living-in-progress.com
Ginger Vieira's upbeat for 'betes sake blog (archives only – no new blogs)

www.ninjabetic.com/
… because it takes being a ninja to live successfully with diabetes

scottsdiabetes.com/
Scott Johnson's struggles, successes, and everything in-between

blog.sstrumello.com/
Scott Strumello's no-holds-barred look at the science of diabetes

sugabetic.wordpress.com/
In the south, you don't have diabetes. You have "the Suga," says Sarah.

thebuttercompartment.com/
Hosted by Lee Ann Thill, diabetes blogger and art therapist

thegirlsguidetodiabetes.com/
Sysy Morales' offbeat observations for girls living with diabetes

thelifeofadiabetic.com/
Chris Stocker's attempt to live a "normal" life with diabetes

tobesugarfree.com/
Christopher Snider says, what good is an incurable disease if you can't share it?

ORGANIZATIONAL SUPPORT

For those in need of resources to cope with the rigors of life with diabetes, as well as those looking to give something back, a number of specialized organizations are ready to take your call:

American Association of Diabetes Educators (AADE)
800-338-3633 www.aadenet.org

American Association of Kidney Patients
800-749-2257 www.aakp.org

American Chronic Pain Association
800 533-3231 www.theacpa.org

American Diabetes Association (ADA)
800-232-3472 www.diabetes.org

American Dietetic Association (also... ADA)
800-877-1600   www.eatright.org

American Foundation for the Blind
800-232-5463   http://www.afb.org/default.aspx

American Heart Association
800-242-8721   http://www.heart.org/HEARTORG/

Amputee Coalition of America
888-267-5669   www.amputee-coalition.org

Celiac Society
www.celiacsociety.com

Celiac Sprue Association/USA
402-558-0600   www.csaceliacs.org

Diabetes Camping Association (DCA)
256-883-2556   www.diabetescamps.org

Friends With Diabetes (Jewish)
845-352-7532   www.friendswithdiabetes.org

International Association for Medical Assistance to Travelers (IAMAT)
716-754-4883   www.iamat.org

Gluten Intolerance Group of North America
206-246-6652   www.gluten.net

Jewish Diabetes Association (JDA)
718-787-4532   www.jewishdiabetes.org

Juvenile Diabetes Research Foundation (JDRF)
800-533-2873   www.jdrf.org

National Center on Physical Activity and Disability
www.ncpad.org

National Federation of the Blind Materials Resource Center
410-659-9314   www.nfb.org

National Kidney Foundation
800-622-9010   www.kidney.org

National Institute of Dental and Craniofacial Research
301-402-7364   www.nidcr.nih.gov

Natl. Institute of Diabetes, Digestive & Kidney Diseases
www.niddk.nih.gov/

National Library Service for the Blind and Physically Handicapped
800-424-8567   www.lcweb.loc.gov/nls

Neuropathy Association
800-247-6968   www.neuropathy.org

National Diabetes Education Program
800-GET-LEVEL
www.niddk.nih.gov/health/diabetes/ndep/ndep.htm

National Diabetes Information Clearinghouse
800-860-8747
www.niddk.nih.gov/health/diabetes/ndc.htmm

National Institute of Diabetes and Digestive and Kidney Diseases
301-496-3583   http://www2.niddk.nih.gov/

National Institute of Health
301-496-4261   www.nih.gov

Taking Control of Your Diabetes (TCOYD)
www.tcoyd.org;

TrialNet
http://www.diabetestrialnet.org/;
e-mail: trialnetinfo@epi.usf.edu

FINANCIAL RESOURCES

A number of programs are in place to help offset the cost of diabetes care.

Medicare is a government-sponsored program for people over age 65 as well as younger people with serious health problems such as kidney failure. Medicare covers blood glucose monitors, test strips, lancets, insulin pumps/supplies, therapeutic shoes, glaucoma screenings, flu and pneumonia vaccines, and limited counseling by some registered dietitians and Certified Diabetes Educators. Medicare Part D provides prescription drug benefits for items such as insulin and oral diabetes medications. For eligibility information, call the Centers for Medicare and Medicaid Services at 1-800-633-4227 or visit www.medicare.gov.

Medicare also offers a database of public and private **prescription drug assistance programs** at http://www. medicare.gov/part-d/index.html. The Washington-DC based Cost Containment Research Institute(202-318-0770) has published a book on free and low-cost medications, available online at Amazon.com: http://www.amazon.com/Free-Cost-Prescription-Drugs-Edition/dp/0974294101; Another web site, www.needymeds.com, provides up-to-date information on nearly 200 patient assistance programs run by drug manufacturers.

Medicaid is a health assistance program sponsored by each individual state. Eligibility is based on your income level. Medicaid recipients may qualify for full or partial coverage for select types of diabetes medications and blood glucose monitors/strips. For information, contact the Department of Human Services in the "government" pages of your phone book.

CHIP is the Children's Health Insurance Program provided by each state. It is for children whose families earn too much to qualify for Medicaid but too little to afford private health insurance. For information, call 877-543-7669 or visit www.insurekidsnow.gov.

PCIP is the pre-existing condition insurance plan, established by the Affordable Care Act, and administered by the U.S. Department of Health and Human Services. It provides a health coverage option for children and adults who have been locked out of the insurance market because of a pre-existing health condition. For information or to apply, find your state at www.pcip.gov or call 866-717-5826.

The Bureau of Primary Health Care (also called the Hill-Burton Program) offers professional medical care regardless of insurance status or ability to pay. For a directory of local primary health care centers, call 800-400-2742 or visit www.bphc.hrsa.gov.

The VA (Department of Veteran Affairs) runs hospitals and clinics for veterans who need treatment for service-related ailments and/or financial aid. To find out more about VA health benefits, call 800-827-1000 or visit www.va.gov.

WIC (Women, Infants & Children)—Healthy eating is an essential component of diabetes self-care. Women with pre-existing diabetes who become pregnant, as well as those who develop gestational diabetes, may be eligible for assistance with grocery costs if certain criteria are met. For more information, call WIC Headquarters at 703-305-2746 or visit www.fns.usda.gov/wic.

Together Rx. People who have no prescription coverage and are not eligible for Medicare may be able to obtain a free Together Rx Access Card. Using the card can save you 25 percent to 40 percent on a select list of brand-name and generic drugs/supplies (including insulin, oral diabetes medications, meters, and test strips). For qualification information and a list of covered drugs, call 800-444-4106 or visit www.togetherrxaccess.com.

Lilly Cares is a patient assistance program for users of Eli Lilly insulin and other medications. Free insulin is provided by way of coupons supplied to your physician. Lilly Cares is open to legal U.S. residents who fail to qualify for government-sponsored programs, do not have private insurance, and fall below a certain income level. For more information, call 800-545-6962 or visit www.lillycares.com.

Novo Nordisk offers a Patient Assistance Program that provides free insulin, pen needles, and glucagon kits for those who fail to qualify for government-sponsored programs, do not have private insurance, and fall below a certain income level. For more information, call 866-310-7549.

Aventis Pharmaceuticals also offers a Patient Assistance Program that provides free insulin to those who fail to qualify for government-sponsored programs, do not have private insurance, and fall below a certain income level. For more information, call 800-221-4025.

Medtronic, makers of insulin pumps and pump supplies, offers financial assistance for those who use (or are looking to use) insulin pumps. Contact the Charles Ray III Diabetes Foundation at 919-303-6949 or visit charlesray.g12.com.

Glucose Test Strip Manufacturers often provide co-pay cards for users of their blood glucose meters. The co-pay cards either reduce or eliminate co-pays associated with test strip purchases. There are usually no income or insurance eligibility limits. For details, call the toll-free number on the back of your glucose meter.

REMOTE CARE

Nowadays, going to the doctor's office doesn't always mean, literally, going to the doctor's office. More and more, medical practices, including many diabetes clinics, offer remote care for their patients. Individuals who live a great distance from their physician or diabetes educator may be able to go to a local clinic for a video conference with their diabetes specialist. Faxed logsheets, e-mailed reports, and downloaded devices allow for a meaningful face-to-face consultation without actually being in the same room.

Research has shown that remote care is safe, cost effective, and clinically effective. Its use was once limited to remote rural areas, but as insurance companies are catching on to the benefits of remote care, it is growing in popularity—even in suburban and urban communities.

Besides medical appointments, remote care can be used to obtain essential diabetes education and interact with a Certified Diabetes Educator. While some health insurance plans still require in-person visits, others are willing to reimburse for care provided by phone or through the Internet.

Some companies and organizations are providing care almost exclusively on a remote basis. For example, Fit4D (fit4d.com) is a wellness and fitness coaching service that operates exclusively online. Nutrition and exercise specialists offer consultations for people with diabetes who have weight loss needs, specific sports/fitness goals, or want to improve their diabetes control.

Integrated Diabetes Services (integrateddiabetes.com) features a multidisciplinary team of Certified Diabetes

Educators who counsel insulin users on blood sugar management strategies and teach advanced self-management skills to clients worldwide. Services are available via phone, e-mail, skype, fax, and live chat.

Webinars are also becoming a popular means for obtaining diabetes education. Both Integrated Diabetes Services and Fit4D offer webinars on various topics in diabetes self-care. Internationally, leading diabetes organizations, governments, and major institutions have come to realize that people with diabetes, and not just health professionals, can benefit from the webinar style of teaching. Check the specific web site for your preferred organizations to find out about webinar offerings.

Index

Vitamin D supplementation, 32

W
WaveSense Diabetes Manager, 91, 112
Web-based resources, for self-
    management
  Diabetes Online Community, 132
  social networking, 131
  specialized blogs and web sites
    childrenwithdiabetes.com, 133
    closeconcerns.com, 133
    Diabetes Advocates, 132
    Diabetes Blogs, 134
    Diabetes Social Media Advocacy,
      132
    Online Diabetes Communities, 132
Weight loss
  diet plans for, 25–26
  "gastric banding" for, 26
  insulin dosage reduction for, 25
White bread, glycemic index score
    of, 30
WIC (Women, Infants & Children), 144
Women with diabetes, potential risks
    faced by, 12–13, 42

X
Xylitol, 127

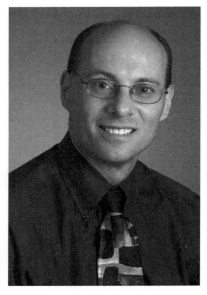

GARY SCHEINER MS, CDE

After earning a Master of Science in Exercise Physiology, Gary Scheiner, MS, CDE, received his diabetes training at the Joslin Diabetes Center. As a Certified Diabetes Educator and person living with diabetes for more than 25 years, he has received numerous awards for his work in the fields of diabetes care and self-management teaching.

Scheiner has written six books and hundreds of articles on various topics in diabetes wellness. Additionally, he teaches the art and science of blood glucose balancing to people throughout the world from his private practice in Wynnewood, Pennsylvania. A dedicated husband and father of five, he enjoys exercising (especially basketball, bicycling, and kickboxing) and cheering on his local Philadelphia sports teams.